The Ultimate Dash Recipes Guide for Beginners

The Perfect Lunch Cookbook to Eat Delicious and Healthy Food for Every Beginner

Maya Wilson

Table of contents

Enjoyable Spinach and Bean Medley

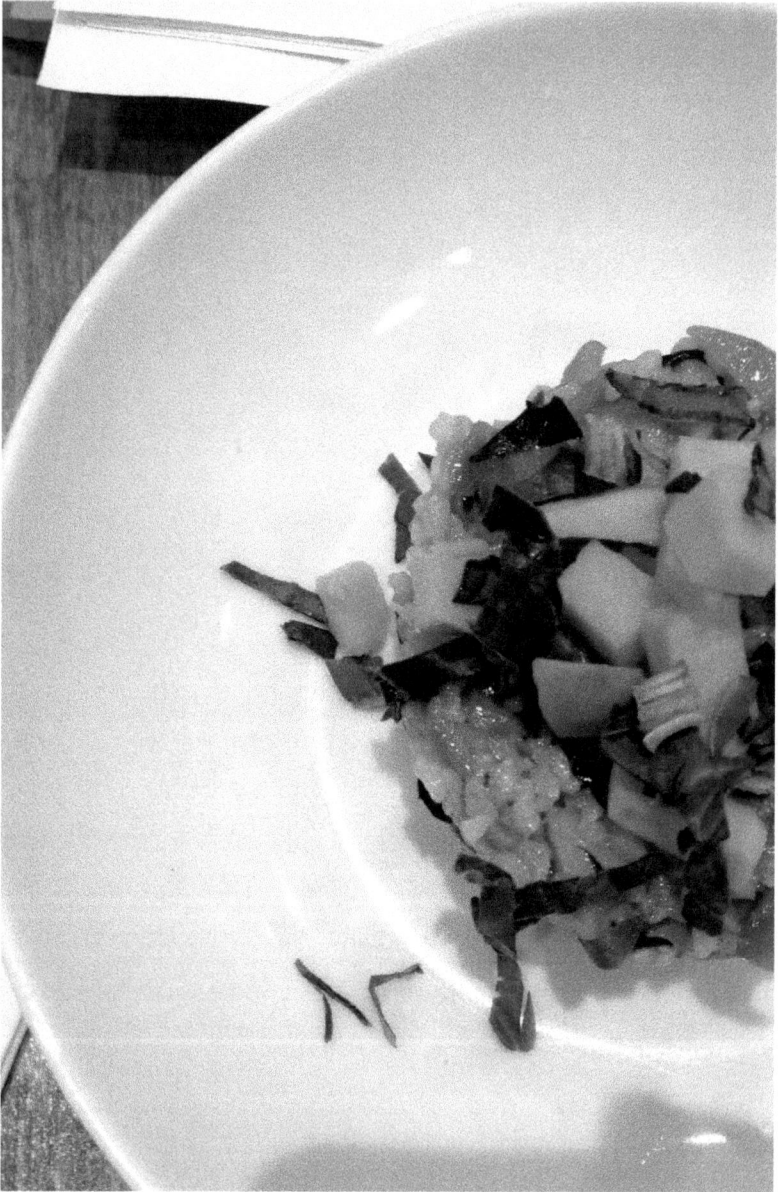

Serving: 4

Prep Time: 10 minutes

Cooking Time: 4 hours

Ingredients:

- 5 carrots, sliced

- 1 ½ cups great northern beans, dried

- 2 garlic cloves, minced

- 1 yellow onion, chopped

- Pepper to taste

- ½ teaspoon oregano, dried

- 5 ounces baby spinach

- 4 ½ cups low sodium veggie stock

- 2 teaspoons lemon peel, grated

- 3 tablespoon lemon juice

How To:

1.   Add beans, onion, carrots, garlic, oregano and stock to your Slow Cooker.

2.   Stir well.
3.   Place lid and cook on HIGH for 4 hours.
4.   Add spinach, juice and lemon rind .
5.   Stir and let it sit for five minutes.
6.   Divide between serving platters and enjoy!

Nutrition (Per Serving)

Calories: 219

Fat: 8g

Carbohydrates: 14g

Protein: 8g

Tantalizing Cauliflower and Dill Mash

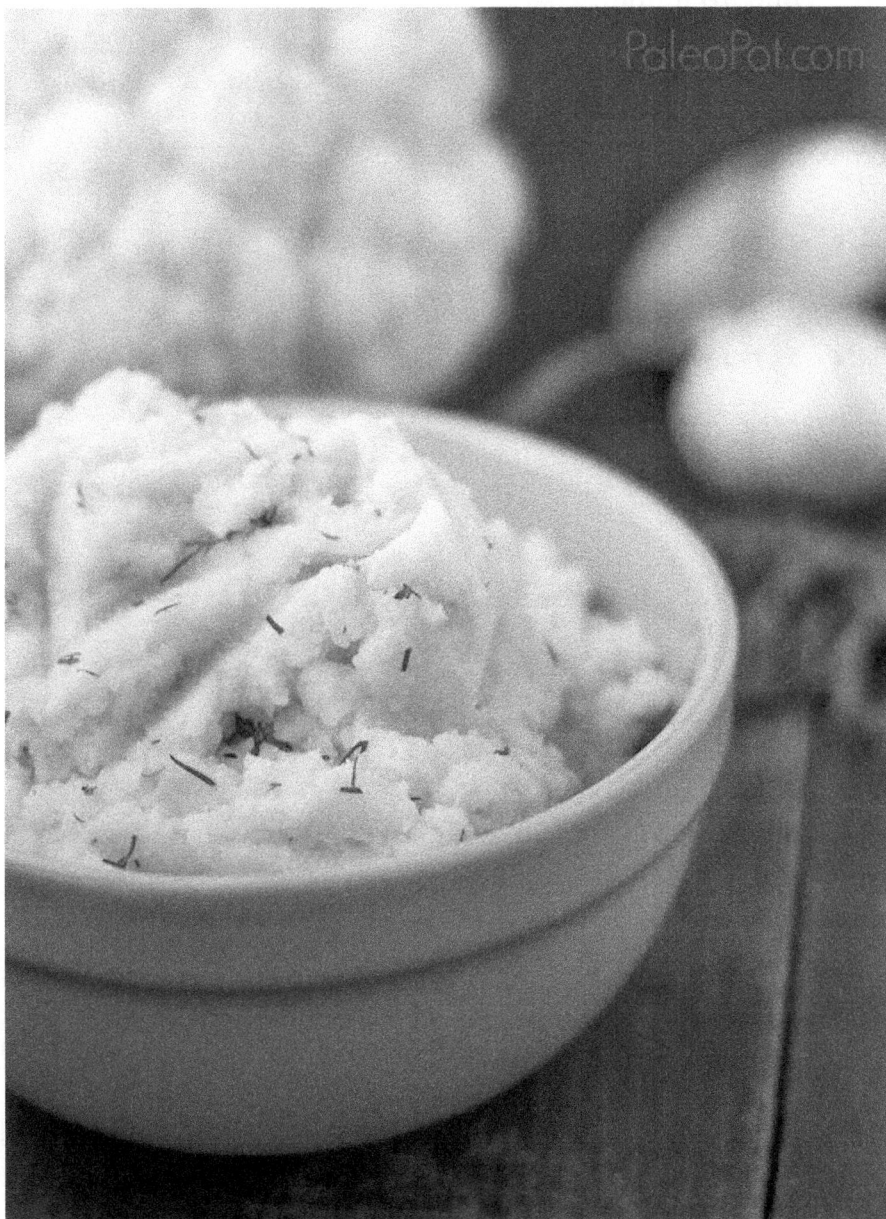

Serving: 6

Prep Time: 10 minutes

Cooking Time: 6 hours

Ingredients:

- 1 cauliflower head, florets separated

- 1/3 cup dill, chopped

- 6 garlic cloves

- 2 tablespoons olive oil

- Pinch of black pepper

How To:

1.   Add cauliflower to Slow Cooker.

2.   Add dill, garlic and water to hide them. 3. Place lid and cook on HIGH for five hours.
3.   Drain the flowers.
4.   Season with pepper and add oil, mash using potato masher.
5.   Whisk and serve.
6.   Enjoy!

Nutrition (Per Serving)

Calories: 207

Fat: 4g

Carbohydrates: 14g

Protein: 3g

Secret Asian Green Beans

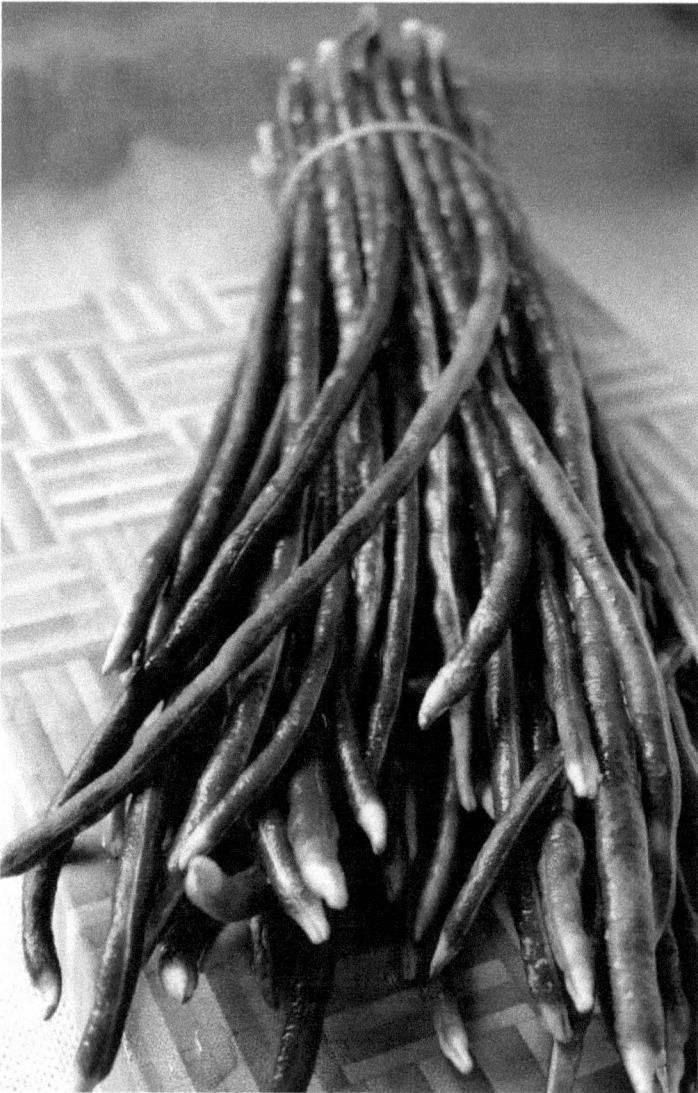

Serving: 10

Prep Time: 10 minutes

Cooking Time: 2 hours

Ingredients:

- 16 cups green beans, halved

- 3 tablespoons olive oil

- ¼ cup tomato sauce, salt-free

- ½ cup coconut sugar

- ¾ teaspoon low sodium soy sauce

- Pinch of pepper

How To:

1.   Add green beans, coconut sugar, pepper spaghetti sauce , soy sauce, oil to your Slow Cooker.

2.   Stir well.
3.   Place lid and cook on LOW for 3 hours.
4.   Divide between serving platters and serve.
5.   Enjoy!

Nutrition (Per Serving)

Calories: 200

Fat: 4g

Carbohydrates: 12g

Protein: 3g

Excellent Acorn Mix

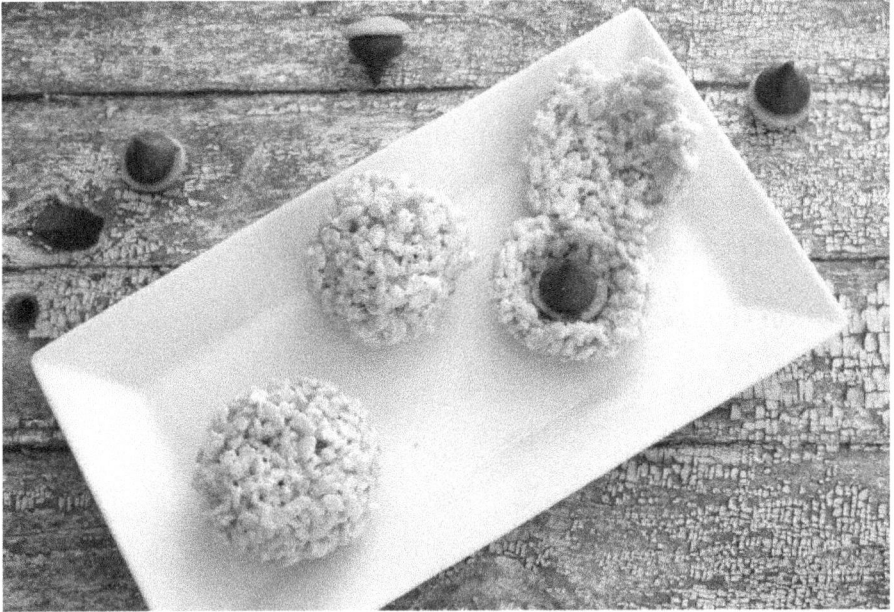

Serving: 10

Prep Time: 10 minutes

Cooking Time: 7 hours

Ingredients:

- 2 acorn squash, peeled and cut into wedges

- 16 ounces cranberry sauce, unsweetened

- ¼ teaspoon cinnamon powder Pepper to taste

How To:

1.   Add acorn wedges to your Slow Cooker.

2.   Add condiment , cinnamon, raisins and pepper.
3.   Stir.
4.   Place lid and cook on LOW for 7 hours.
5.   Serve and enjoy!

Nutrition (Per Serving)

Calories: 200

Fat: 3g

Carbohydrates: 15g

Protein: 2g

Crunchy Almond Chocolate Bars

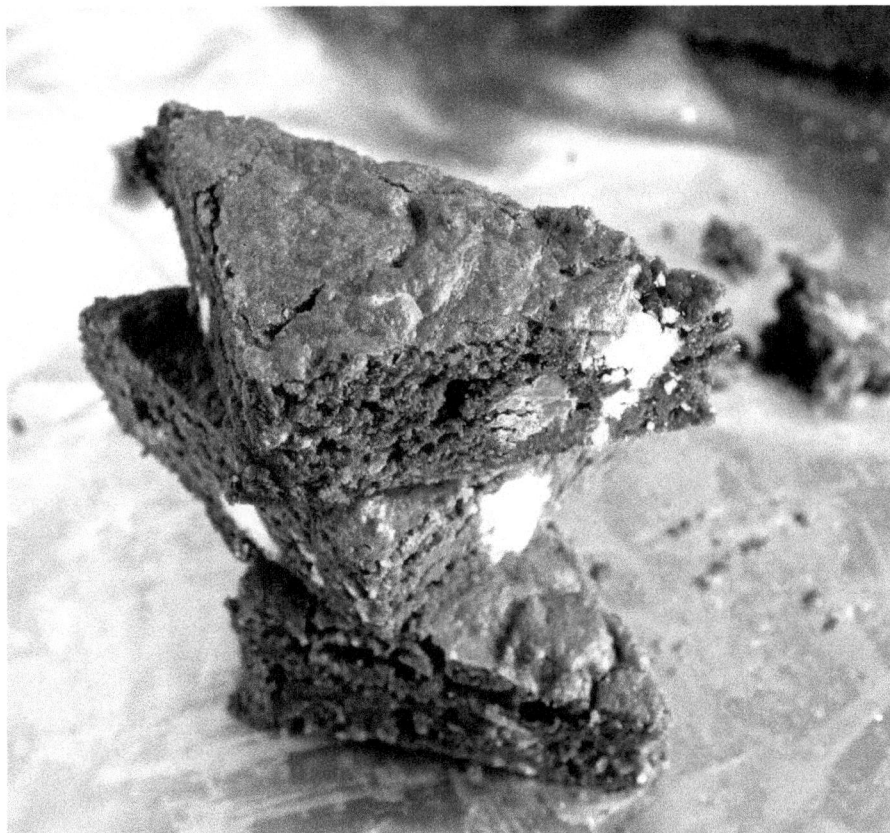

Serving: 12

Prep Time: 10 minutes

Cooking Time: 2 hours 30 minutes

Ingredients:

- 1 egg white

- ¼ cup coconut oil, melted

- 1 cup coconut sugar

- ½ teaspoon vanilla extract

- 1 teaspoon baking powder

- 1 ½ cups almond meal

- ½ cup dark chocolate chips

How To:

1.   Take a bowl and add sugar, oil, vanilla , egg white, almond flour, leaven and blend it well.

2.   Fold in chocolate chips and stir.
3.   Line Slow Cooker with parchment paper.
4.   Grease.
5.   Add the cookie mix and continue bottom.
6.   Place lid and cook on LOW for two hours half-hour .
7.   Take cooking utensil out and let it cool.

8. Cut in bars and enjoy!

Nutrition (Per Serving)

Calories: 200

Fat: 2g

Carbohydrates: 13g

Protein: 6g

Lettuce and Chicken Platter

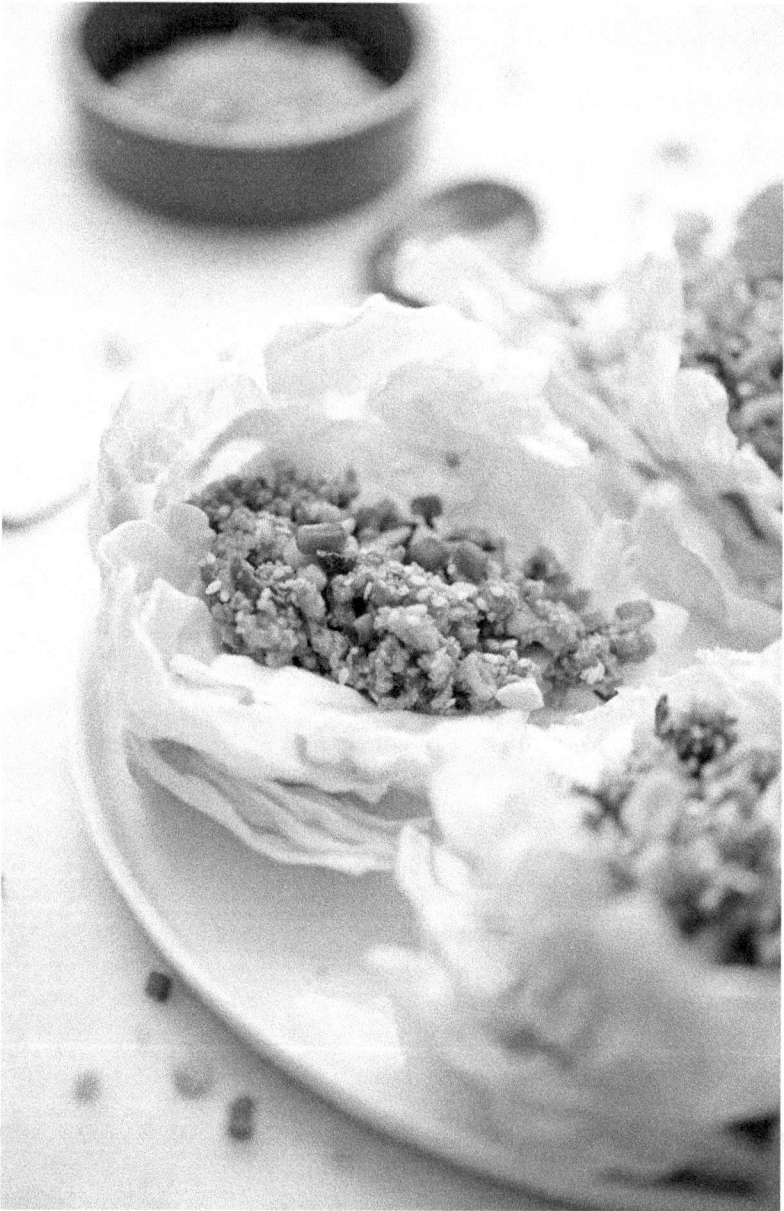

Serving: 6

Prep Time: 10 minutes

Cook Time: nil

Ingredients:

- 2 cups chicken, cooked and coarsely chopped ½ head ice berg lettuce, sliced and chopped 1 celery rib, chopped

- 1 medium apple, cut

- ½ red bell pepper, deseeded and chopped 6-7 green olives, pitted and halved 1 red onion, chopped

- For dressing

- 1 tablespoon raw honey

- 2 tablespoons lemon juice

- Salt and pepper to taste

How To:

1. Cut the vegetables and transfer them to your Salad Bowl.

2.   Add olives.
3.   Chop the cooked chicken and transfer to your Salad bowl.
4.   Prepare dressing by mixing the ingredients listed under Dressing.

5.   Pour the dressing into the Salad bowl.
6.   Toss and enjoy!

Nutrition (Per Serving)

Calories: 296

Fat: 21g

Carbohydrates: 9g

Protein: 18g

Greek Lemon Chicken Bowl

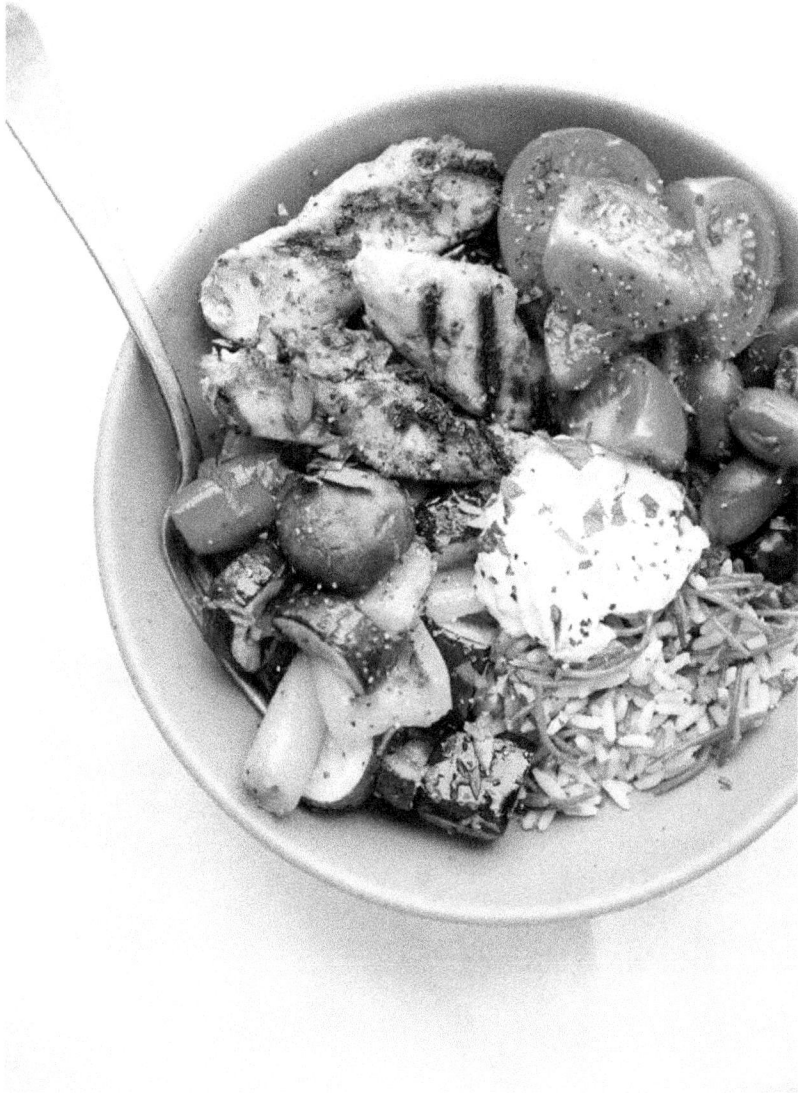

Serving: 6

Prep Time: 10 minutes

Cook Time: 15 minutes

Ingredients:

- 2 cups chicken, cooked and chopped

- 2 cans chicken broth, fat free

- 2 medium carrots, chopped

- ¼ teaspoon pepper

- 2 tablespoons parsley, snipped

- ¼ cup lemon juice

- 1 can cream chicken soup, fat free, low sodium ½ cup onion, chopped

- 1 garlic clove, minced

How To:

1. Take a pot and add all the ingredients except parsley into it.

2. Season with salt and pepper.
3. Bring the combination to a overboil medium-high heat.

4. Reduce the warmth and simmer for quarter-hour .
5. Garnish with parsley.
6. Serve hot and enjoy!

Nutrition (Per Serving)

Calories: 520

Fat: 33g

Carbohydrates: 31g

Protein: 30g

Chilled Chicken, Artichoke and Zucchini Platter

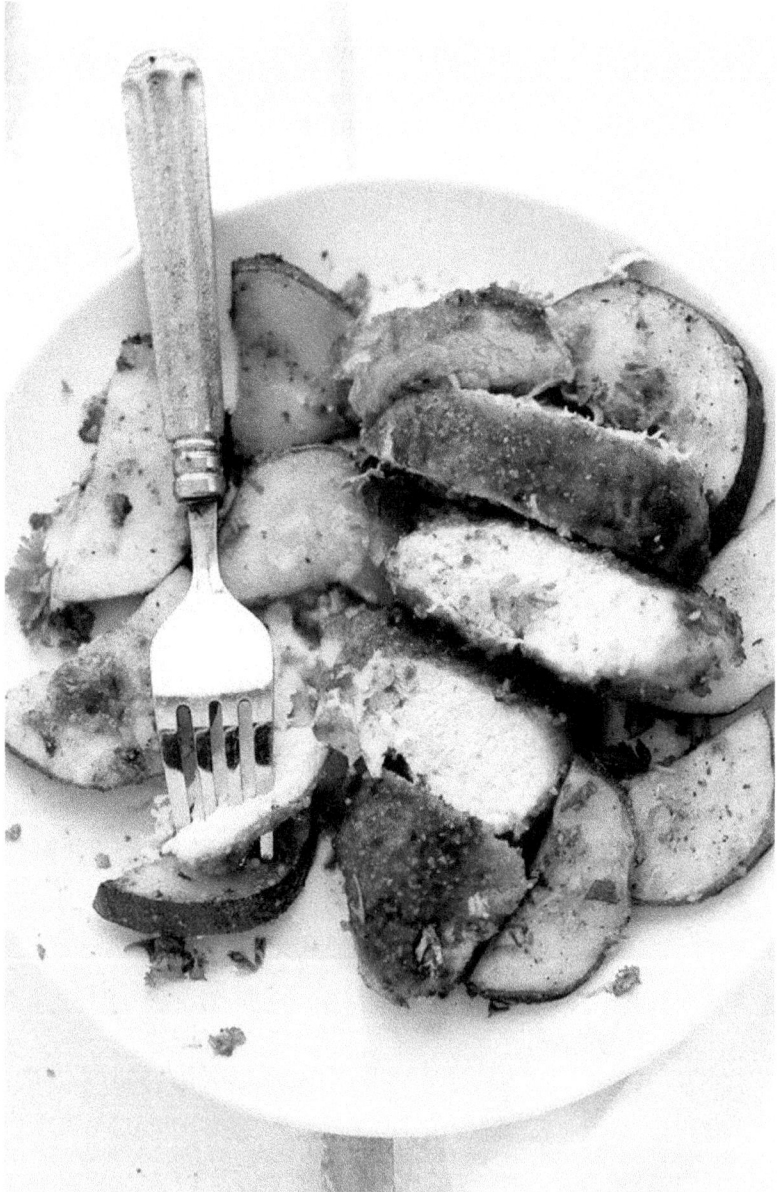

Serving: 4

Prep Time: 10 minutes

Cook Time: 5 minutes

Ingredients:

- 2 medium chicken breasts, cooked and cut into 1-inch cubes ¼ cup extra virgin olive oil

- 2 cups artichoke hearts, drained and roughly chopped

- 3 large zucchini, diced/cut into small rounds

- 1 can (15 ounce) chickpeas

- 1 cup Kalamata olives

- ½ teaspoon Fresh ground black pepper

- ½ teaspoon Italian seasoning

- ¼ cup parmesan, grated

How To:

1.   Take an outsized skillet and place it over medium heat, heat up vegetable oil .

2.   Add zucchini and sauté for five minutes, season with salt and pepper.
3.   Remove from heat and add all the listed ingredients to the skillet.

4.   Stir until combined.
5.   Transfer to glass container and store.
6.   Serve and enjoy!

Nutrition (Per Serving)

Calories: 457

Fat: 22g

Carbohydrates: 30g

Protein: 24g

Chicken and Carrot Stew

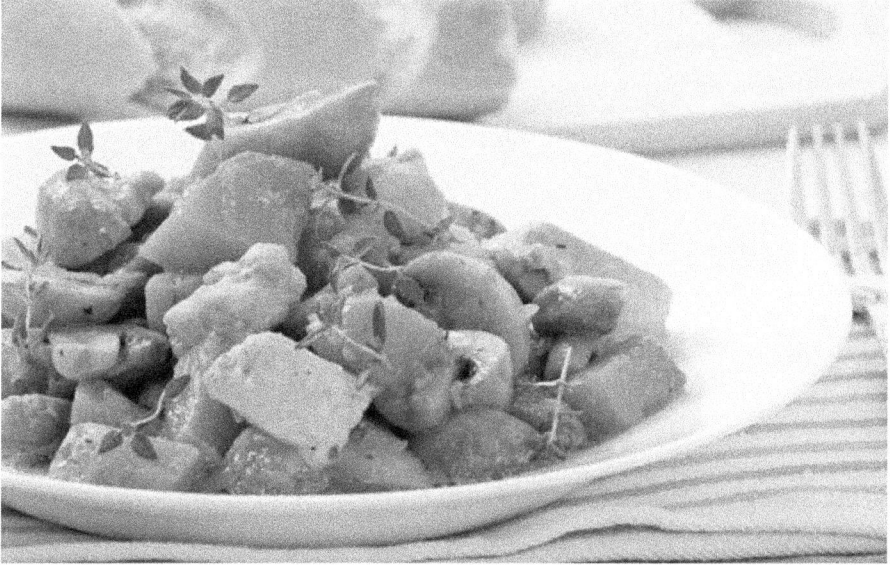

Serving: 6

Prep Time: 15 minutes

Cook Time: 6 hours

Ingredients:

- 4 chicken breasts, boneless and cubed

- 2 cups chicken broth

- 1 cup tomatoes, chopped

- 3 cups carrots, peeled and cubed

- 1 teaspoon thyme dried

- 1 cup onion, chopped

- 2 garlic clove, minced

- Pepper to taste

How To:

1.   Add all the ingredients to the Slow Cooker.

2.   Stir and shut the lid.
3.   Cook for six hours.
4.   Serve hot and enjoy!

Nutrition (Per Serving)

Calories: 182

Fat: 4g

Carbohydrates: 10g

Protein: 39g

Tasty Spinach Pie

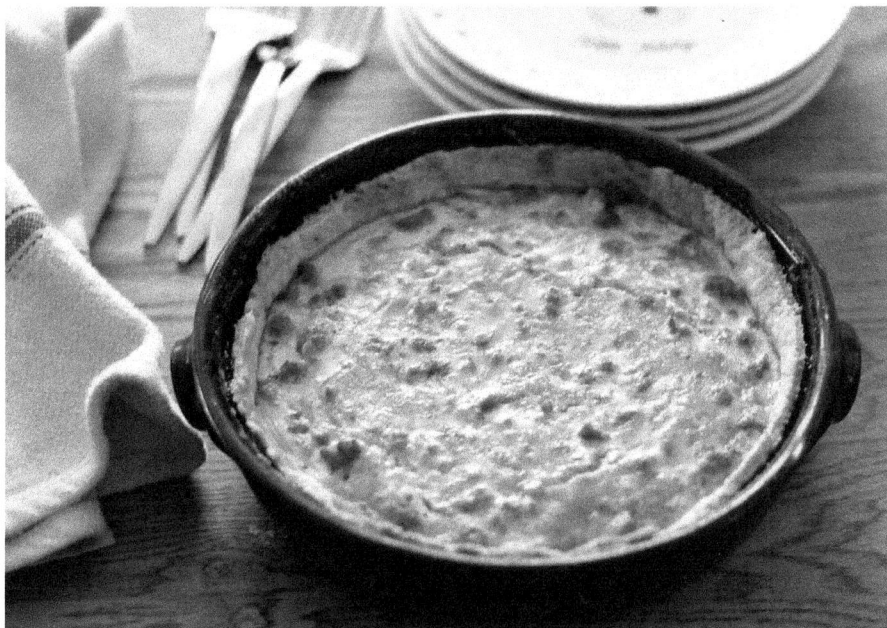

Serving: 2

Prep Time: 10 minutes

Cooking Time: 4 hours

Ingredients:

- 10 ounces spinach

- 2 cups baby Bella mushrooms, chopped

- 1 red bell pepper, chopped

- 1 ½ cups low-fat cheese, shredded

- 8 whole eggs

- 1 cup coconut cream

- 2 tablespoons chives, chopped

- Pinch of pepper

- ½ cup almond flour

- ¼ teaspoon baking soda

How To:

1.   Take a bowl and add eggs, coconut milk , chives, pepper and whisk well.

2.   Add almond flour, bicarbonate of soda , cheese, mushrooms bell pepper, spinach and toss well.
3.   Grease your cooker and transfer mix to the Slow Cooker.
4.   Place lid and cook on LOW for 4 hours.
5.   Slice and enjoy!

Nutrition (Per Serving)

Calories: 201

Fat: 6g

Carbohydrates: 8g

Protein: 5g

Mesmerizing Carrot and Pineapple Mix

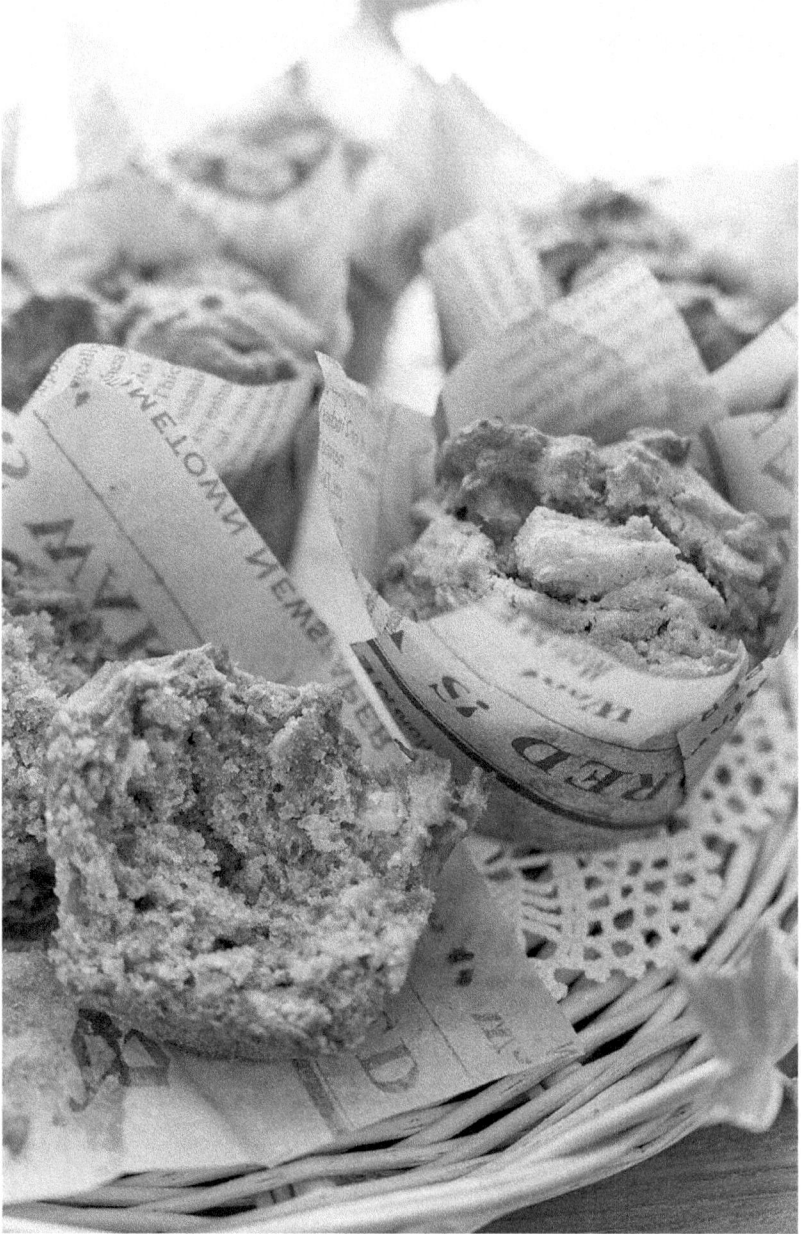

Serving: 10

Prep Time: 10 minutes

Cooking Time: 6 hours

Ingredients:

1 cup raisins 6 cups water

- 23 ounces natural applesauce

- 2 tablespoons stevia

- 2 tablespoons cinnamon powder

- 14 ounces carrots, shredded

- 8 ounces canned pineapple, crushed

- 1 tablespoon pumpkin pie spice

How To:

1.	Add carrots, applesauce, raisins, stevia, cinnamon, pineapple, pie spice to your Slow Cooker and gently stir.

2.	Place lid and cook on LOW for six hours .
3.	Serve and enjoy!

Nutrition (Per Serving)

Calories: 179

Fat: 5g

Carbohydrates: 15g

Protein: 4g

Blackberry Chicken Wings

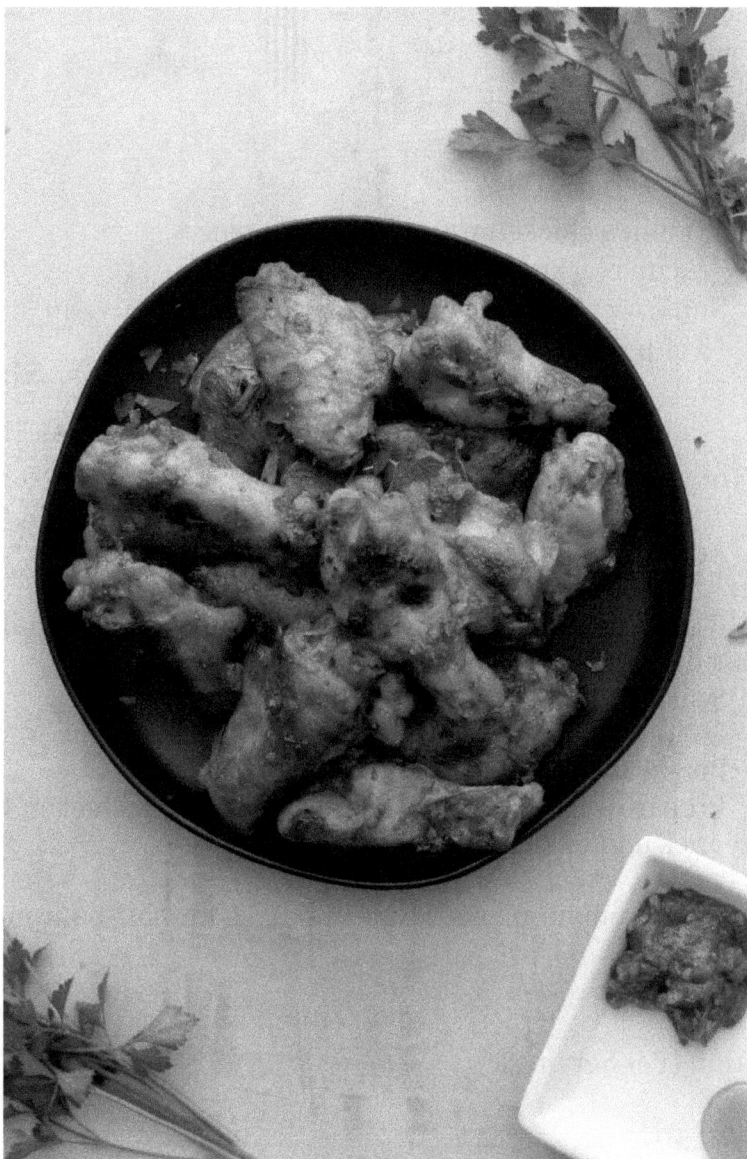

Serving: 4

Prep Time: 35 minutes

Cook Time: 50minutes

Ingredients:

- 3 pounds chicken wings, about 20 pieces
- ½ cup blackberry chipotle jam
- Sunflower seeds and pepper to taste
- ½ cup water

How To:

1. Add water and jam to a bowl and blend well.

2. Place chicken wings during a zip bag and add two-thirds of the marinade.
3. Season with sunflower seeds and pepper.
4. Let it marinate for half-hour .
5. Pre-heat your oven to 400 degrees F.
6. Prepare a baking sheet and wire rack, place chicken wings in wire rack and bake for quarter-hour .

7. Brush remaining marinade and bake for half-hour more.

8. Enjoy!

Nutrition (Per Serving)

Calories: 502

Fat: 39g

Carbohydrates: 01.8g

Protein: 34g

Generous Lemon Dredged Broccoli

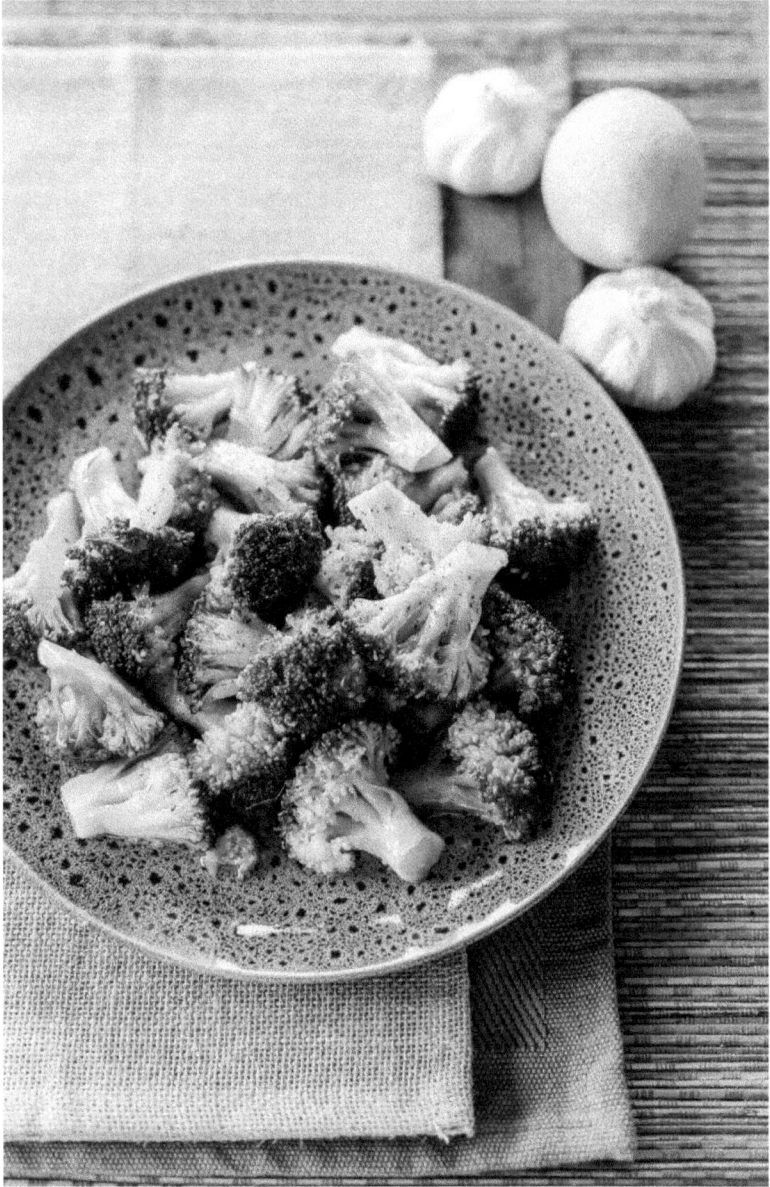

Serving: 4

Prep Time: 10 minutes

Cook Time: 15 minutes

Ingredients:

- 2 heads broccoli, separated into florets

- 2 teaspoons extra virgin olive oil

- 1 teaspoon sunflower seeds

- ½ teaspoon pepper

- 1 garlic clove, minced

- ½ teaspoon lemon juice

How To:

1.   Pre-heat your oven to a temperature of 400 degrees F.

2.   Take an outsized sized bowl and add broccoli florets with some extra virgin vegetable oil , pepper, sea sunflower seeds and garlic.

3.   Spread the broccoli call at one even layer on a fine baking sheet.

4.   Bake in your pre-heated oven for about 15-20 minutes until the florets are soft enough to be pierced with a fork.
5.   Squeeze juice over them generously before serving.
6.   Enjoy!

Nutrition (Per Serving)

Calories: 49

Fat: 2g

Carbohydrates: 4g

Protein: 3g

Tantalizing Almond butter Beans

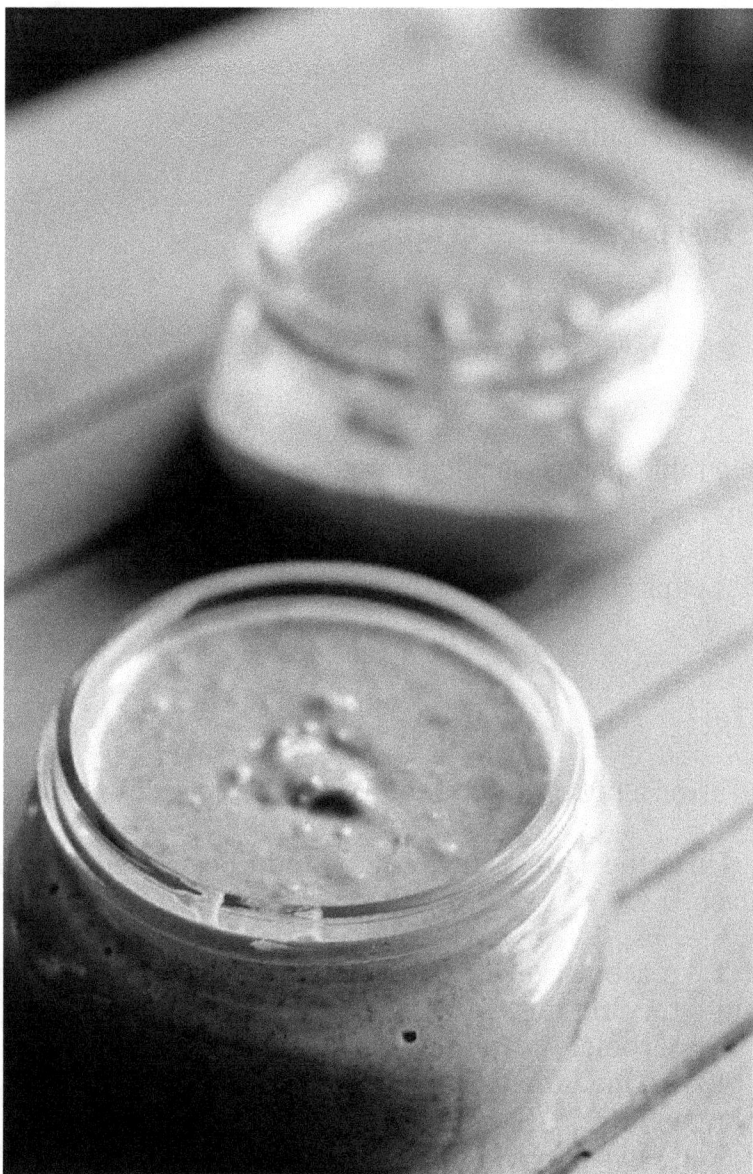

Serving: 4

Prep Time: 5 minutes

Cook Time: 12 minutes

Ingredients:

2 garlic cloves, minced

- Red pepper flakes to taste

- Sunflower seeds to taste

- 2 tablespoons clarified butter

- 4 cups green beans, trimmed

How To:

1.   Bring a pot of water to boil, with added seeds for taste.

2.   Once the water starts to boil, add beans and cook for 3 minutes.

3.   Take a bowl of drinking water and drain beans, plunge them into the drinking water .
4.   Once cooled, keep them on the side.
5.   Take a medium skillet and place it over medium heat, add ghee and melt.
6.   Add red pepper, sunflower seeds, garlic.
7.   Cook for 1 minute.

8.   Add beans and toss until coated well, cook for 3 minutes.

9.   Serve and enjoy!

Nutrition (Per Serving)

Calories: 93

Fat: 8g

Carbohydrates: 4g

Protein: 2g

Healthy Chicken Cream Salad

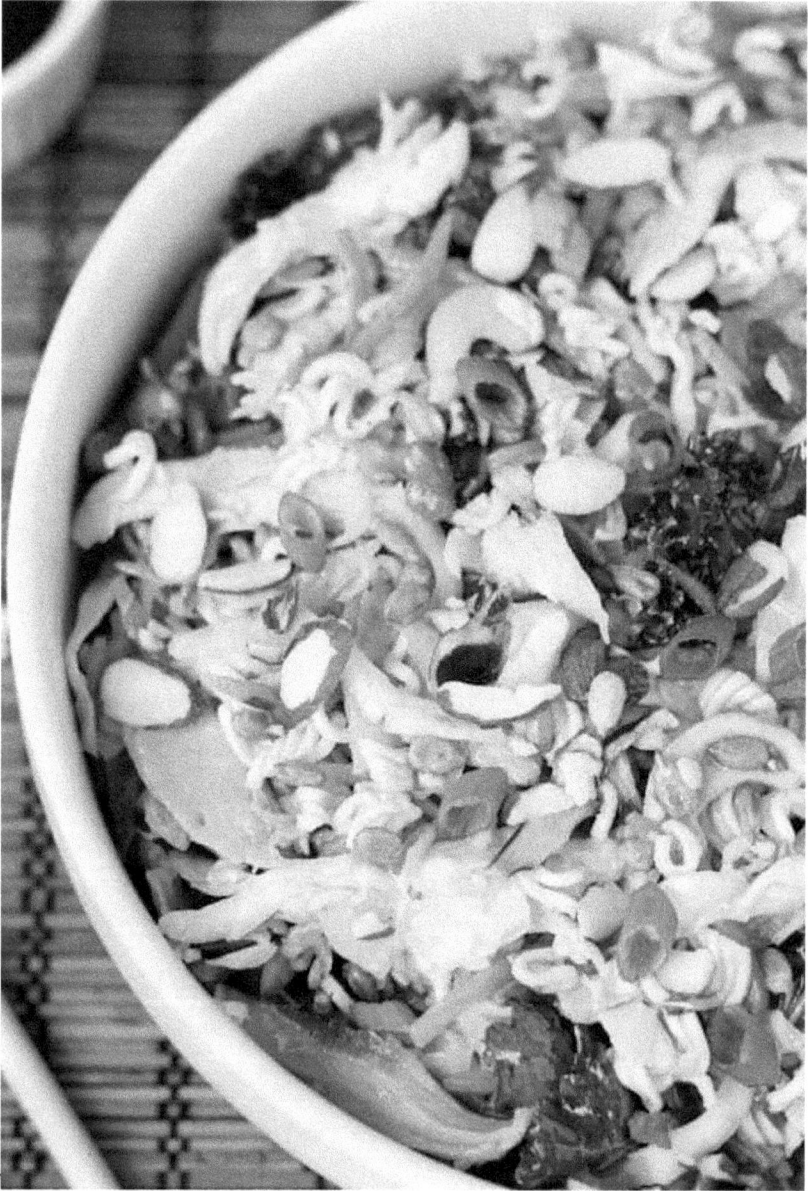

7

Serving: 3

Prep Time: 5 minutes

Cook Time: 50 minutes

Ingredients:

- 2 chicken breasts

- 1 ½ cups low fat cream

- 3 ounces celery

- 2 ounce green pepper, chopped

- ½ ounce green onion, chopped

- ½ cup low fat mayo

- 3 hard-boiled eggs, chopped

How To:

1. Pre-heat your oven to 350 degrees F.

2. Take a baking sheet and place chicken, cover with cream.

3.   Bake for 30-40 minutes.
4.   Take a bowl and blend within the chopped celery, peppers, onions.

5.   Chop the baked chicken into bite-sized portions.
6.   Peel and chop the hard boiled eggs.
7.   Take an outsized salad bowl and blend in eggs, veggies and chicken.
8.   Toss well and serve.
9.   Enjoy!

Nutrition (Per Serving)

Calories: 415

Fat: 24g

Carbohydrates: 4g

Protein: 40g

Generously Smothered Pork Chops

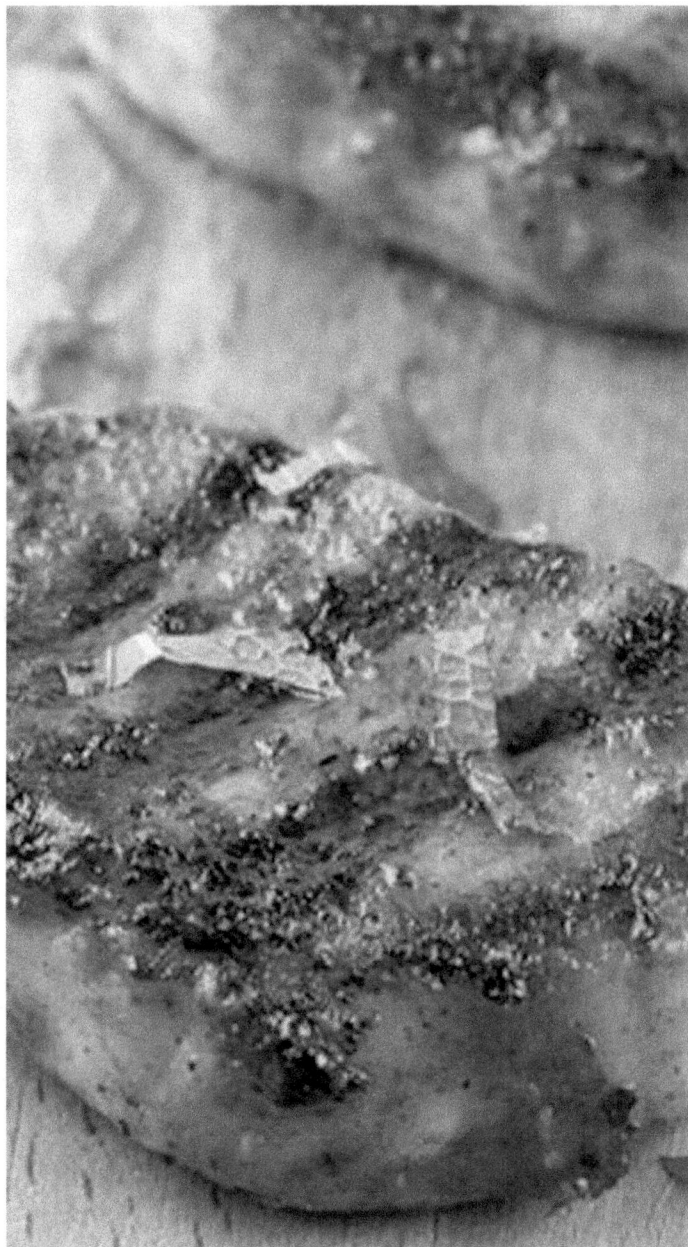

Serving: 4

Prep Time: 10 minutes

Cook Time: 30 minutes

Ingredients:

- 4 pork chops, bone-in

- 2 tablespoons of olive oil

- ¼ cup vegetable broth

- ½ pound Yukon gold potatoes, peeled and chopped 1 large onion, sliced

- 2 garlic cloves, minced

- 2 teaspoon rubbed sage

- 1 teaspoon thyme, ground

- Pepper as needed

How To:

1.   Pre-heat your oven to 350 degrees F.

2.   Take an outsized sized skillet and place it over medium heat.

3.   Add a tablespoon of oil and permit the oil to heat up.

4.   Add pork chops and cook them for 4-5 minutes per side until browned.

5.   Transfer chops to a baking dish.

6.   Pour broth over the chops.

7.   Add remaining oil to the pan and sauté potatoes, onion, garlic for 3-4 minutes.

8.   Take an outsized bowl and add potatoes, garlic, onion, thyme, sage, pepper.

9.   Transfer this mixture to the baking dish (wish pork).

10.   Bake for 20-30 minutes.

11.   Serve and enjoy!

Nutrition (Per Serving)

Calorie: 261

Fat: 10g

Carbohydrates: 1.3g

Protein: 2g

Crazy Lamb Salad

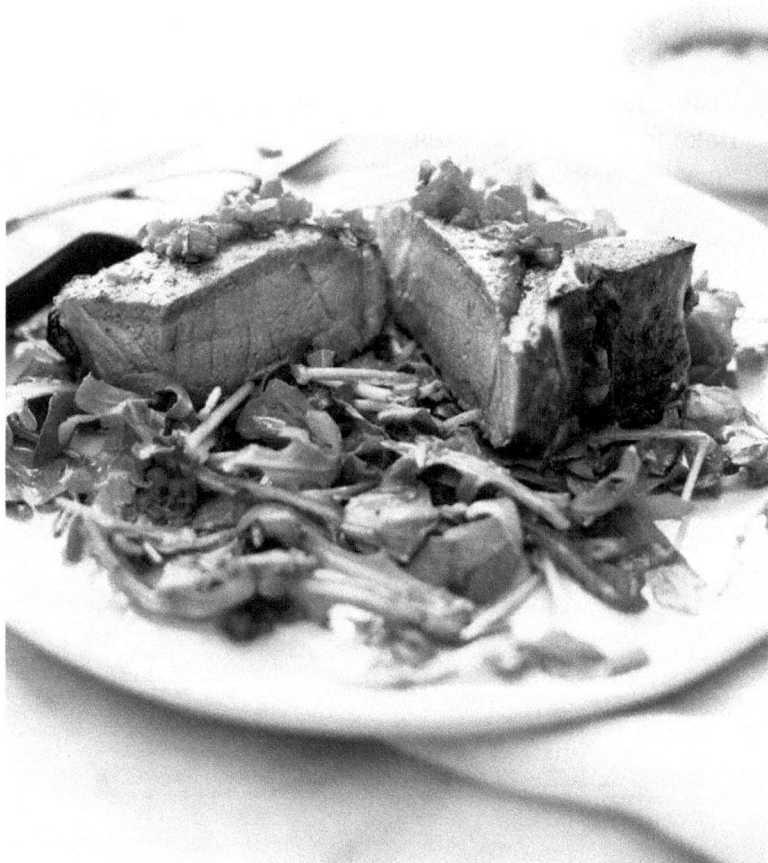

Serving: 4

Prep Time: 10 minutes

Cook Time: 35 minutes

Ingredients:

- 1 tablespoon olive oil

- 3 pound leg of lamb, bone removed, leg butterflied Salt and pepper to taste

- 1 teaspoon cumin

- Pinch of dried thyme

- 2 garlic cloves, peeled and minced For Salad

- 4 ounces feta cheese, crumbled

- ½ cup pecans

- 2 cups spinach

- 1 ½ tablespoons lemon juice

- ¼ cup olive oil

- 1 cup fresh mint, chopped

How To:

1.   Rub lamb with salt and pepper, 1 tablespoon oil, thyme, cumin, minced garlic.

2.   Pre-heat your grill to medium-high and transfer lamb.
3.   Cook for 40 minutes, ensuring to flip it once.
4.   Take a lined baking sheet and spread the pecans.
5.   Toast in oven for 10 minutes at 350 degree F.
6.   Transfer grilled lamb to chopping board and let it cool.
7.   Slice.
8.   Take a salad bowl and add spinach, 1 cup mint, feta cheese, ¼ cup vegetable oil , juice , toasted pecans, salt, pepper and toss well.

9.   Add lamb slices on top.
10.   Serve and enjoy!

Nutrition (Per Serving)

Calories: 334

Fat: 33g

Carbohydrates: 5g

Protein: 7g

Hearty Roasted Cauliflower

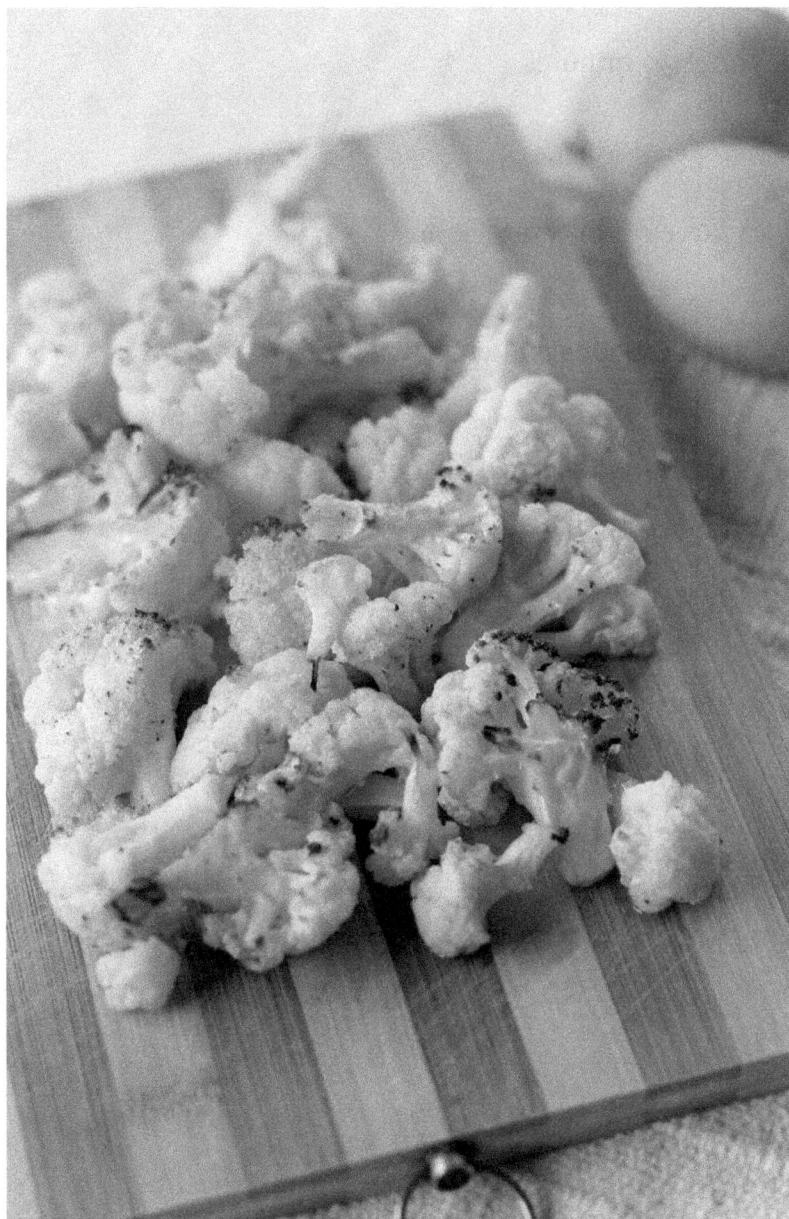

Serving: 8

Prep Time: 5 minutes

Cook Time: 30 minutes

Ingredients:

- 1 large cauliflower head

- 2 tablespoons melted coconut oil

- 2 tablespoons fresh thyme

- 1 teaspoon Celtic sea sunflower seeds

- 1 teaspoon fresh ground pepper

- 1 head roasted garlic

- 2 tablespoons fresh thyme for garnish

How To:

1. Pre-heat your oven to 425 degrees F.
2. Rinse cauliflower and trim, core and sliced.
3. Lay cauliflower evenly on rimmed baking tray.

4. Drizzle copra oil evenly over cauliflower, sprinkle thyme leaves .

5. Season with pinch of sunflower seeds and pepper.
6. Squeeze roasted garlic.
7. Roast cauliflower until slightly caramelized for about half-hour , ensuring to show once.
8. Garnish with fresh thyme leaves.
9. Enjoy!

Nutrition (Per Serving)

Calories: 129

Fat: 11g

Carbohydrates: 6g

Protein: 7g

Cool Cabbage Fried Beef

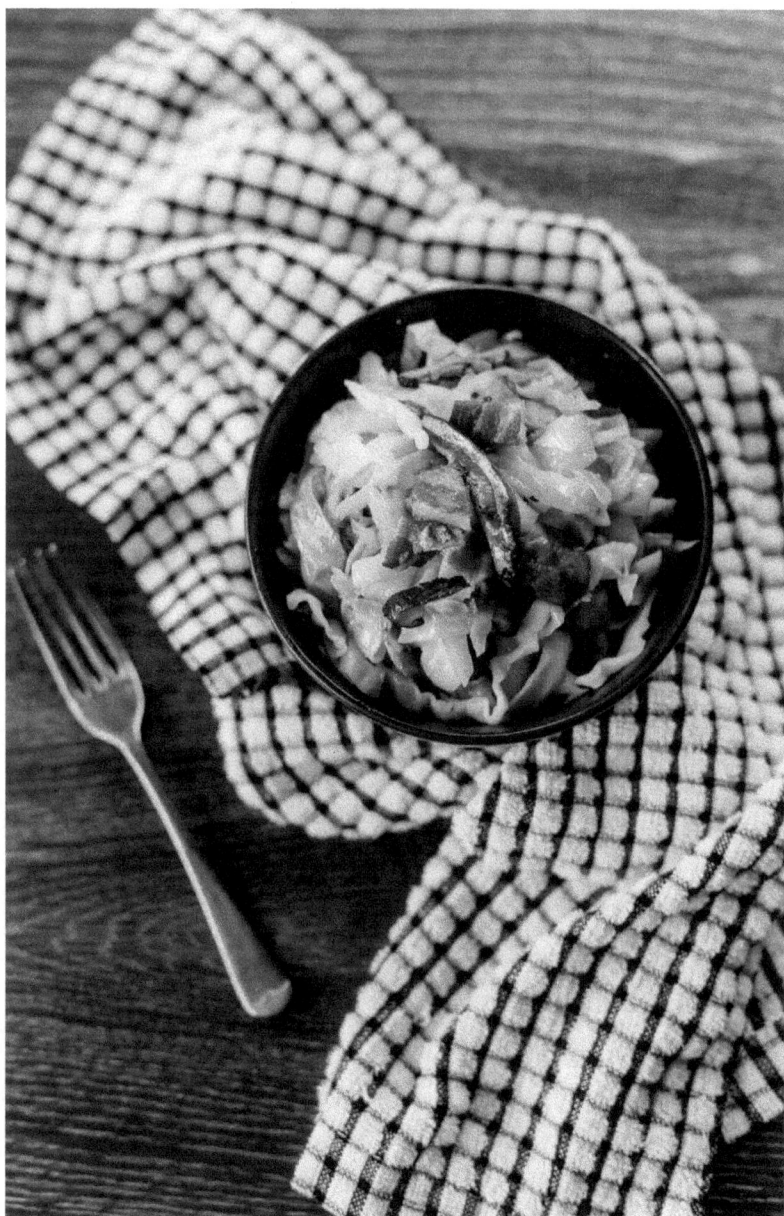

Serving: 4

Prep Time: 5 minutes

Cook Time: 15 minutes

Ingredients:

- 1-pound beef, ground and lean

- ½ pound bacon

- 1 onion

- 1 garlic clove, minced

- ½ head cabbage

- pepper to taste

How To:

1. Take skillet and place it over medium heat.

2. Add chopped bacon, beef and onion until slightly browned.
3. Transfer to a bowl and keep it covered.

4.   Add minced garlic and cabbage to the skillet and cook until slightly browned.
5.   Return the bottom beef mix to the skillet and simmer for 3-5 minutes over low heat.
6.   Serve and enjoy!

Nutrition (Per Serving)

Calories: 360

Fat: 22g

Net Carbohydrates: 5g

Protein: 34g

Fennel and Figs Lamb

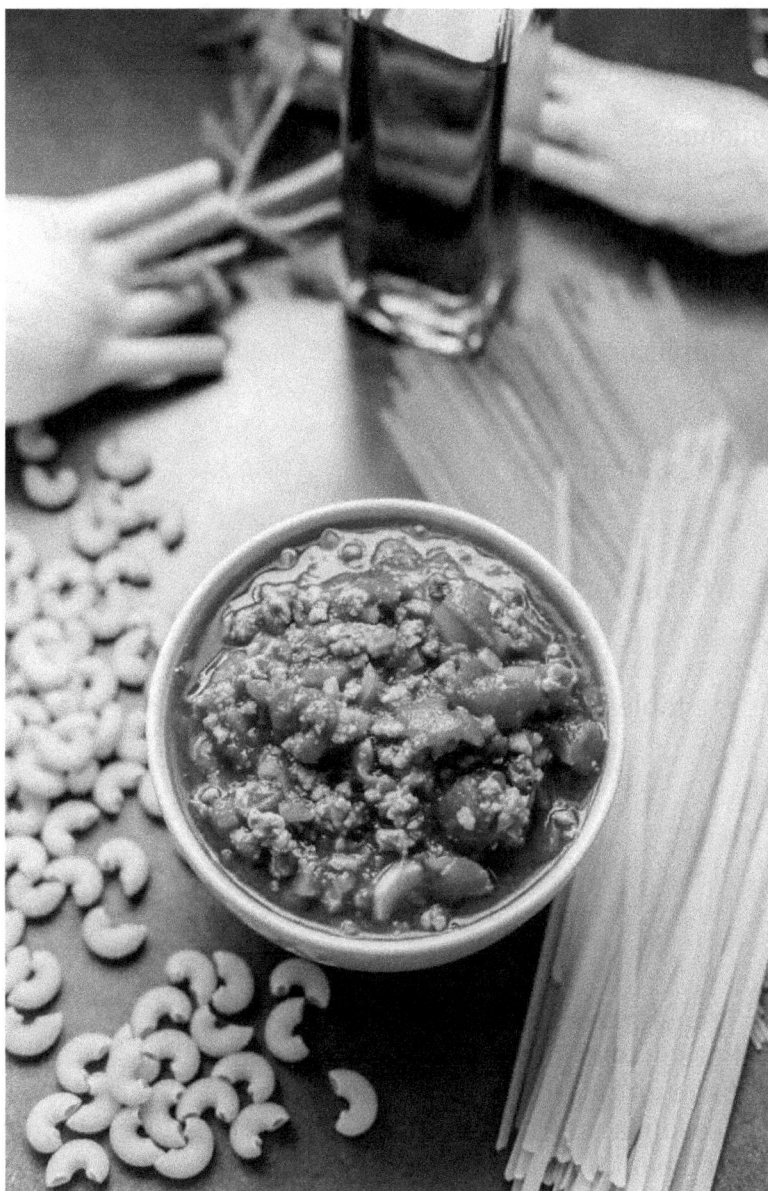

Serving: 2

Prep Time: 10 minutes

Cook Time: 40 minutes

Ingredients:

- 6 ounces lamb racks 1 fennel bulbs, sliced pepper to taste

- 1 tablespoon olive oil

- 2 figs, cut in half

- 1/8 cup apple cider vinegar

- 1/2 tablespoon swerve

How To:

1.   Take a bowl and add fennel, figs, vinegar, swerve, oil and toss.

2.   Transfer to baking dish.
3.   Season with sunflower seeds and pepper.
4.   Bake for quarter-hour at 400 degrees F.
5.   Season lamb with sunflower seeds and pepper and transfer to a heated pan over medium-high heat.
6.   Cook for a couple of minutes.

7.   Add lamb to the baking dish with fennel and bake for 20 minutes.

8.   Divide between plates and serve.

9.   Enjoy!

Nutrition (Per Serving)

Calories: 230

Fat: 3g

Carbohydrates: 5g

Protein: 10g

Black Berry Chicken Wings

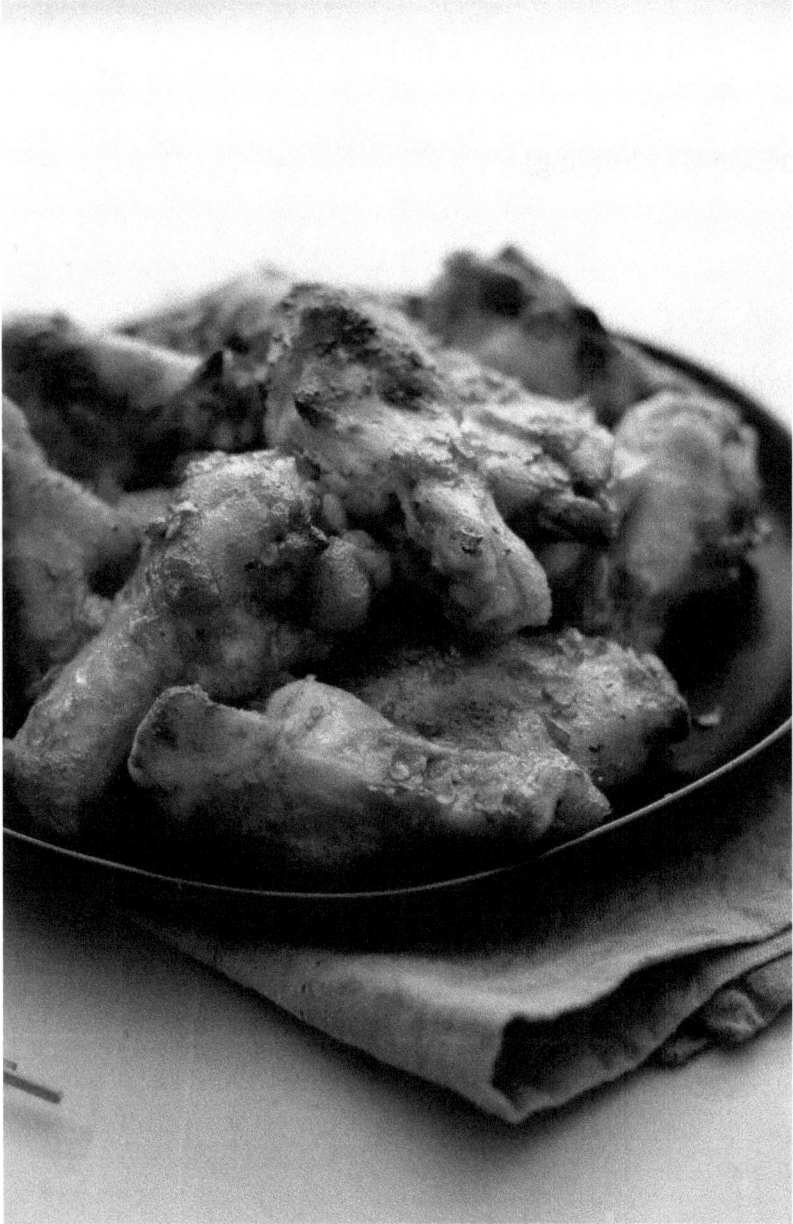

Serving: 4

Prep Time: 35 minutes

Cook Time: 50minutes

Ingredients:

- 3 pounds chicken wings, about 20 pieces ½ cup blackberry chipotle jam Pepper to taste

- ½ cup water

How To:

1.   Add water and jam to a bowl and blend well.

2.   Place chicken wings during a zip bag and add two-thirds of marinade.
3.   Season with pepper.
4.   Let it marinate for half-hour .
5.   Pre-heat your oven to 400 degrees F.
6.   Prepare a baking sheet and wire rack, place chicken wings in wire rack and bake for quarter-hour .
7.   Brush remaining marinade and bake for half-hour more.
8.   Enjoy!

Nutrition (Per Serving)

Calories: 502

Fat: 39g

Carbohydrates: 01.8g

Protein: 34g

Mushroom and Olive "Mediterranean" Steak

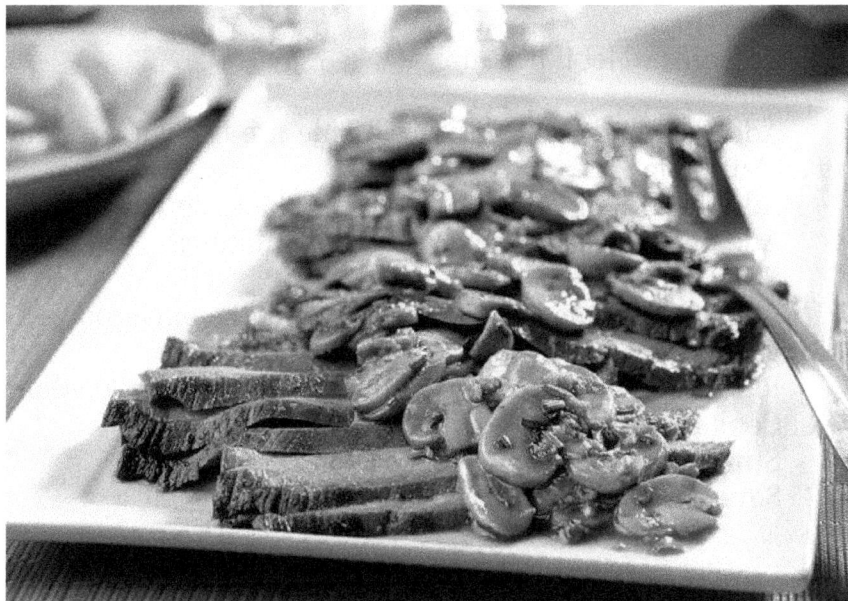

Serving: 2

Prep Time: 10 minutes

Cook Time: 14 minutes

Ingredients:

How To:

Take an outsized sized skillet and place it over medium-high heat.

1.   Add oil and let it heat up.

2.   Add beef and cook until each side are browned, remove beef and drain fat.
3.   Add the remainder of the oil to the skillet and warmth .
4.   Add onions, garlic and cook for 2-3 minutes.
5.   Stir well.
6.   Add mushrooms, olives and cook until the mushrooms are thoroughly done.
7.   Return the meat to the skillet and reduce heat to medium.
8.   Cook for 3-4 minutes (covered).
9.   Stir in parsley.
10.   Serve and enjoy!

Nutrition (Per Serving)

Calories: 386

Fat: 30g

Carbohydrates: 11g

Protein: 21g

Hearty Chicken Fried Rice

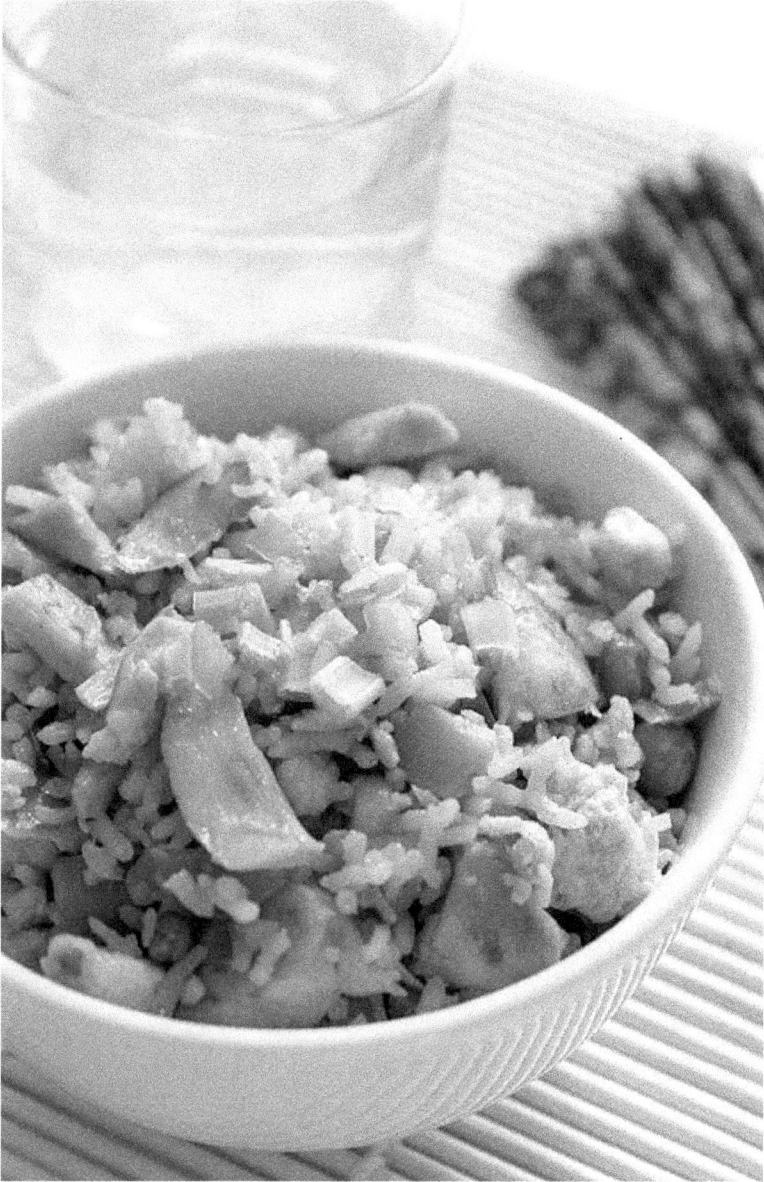

Serving: 4

Prep Time: 10 minutes

Cook Time: 12 minutes

Ingredients:

- 1 teaspoon olive oil

- 4 large egg whites

- 1 onion, chopped

- 2 garlic cloves, minced

- 12 ounces skinless chicken breasts, boneless, cut into ½ inch cubes

- ½ cup carrots, chopped

- ½ cup frozen green peas

- 2 cups long grain brown rice, cooked

- 3 tablespoons soy sauce, low sodium

How To:

1. Coat skillet with oil, place it over medium-high heat.

2. Add egg whites and cook until scrambled .
3. Sauté onion, garlic and chicken breasts for six minutes.

4. Add carrots, peas and keep cooking for 3 minutes.
5. Stir in rice, season with soy .
6. Add cooked egg whites, stir for 3 minutes.
7. Enjoy!

Nutrition (Per Serving)

Calories: 353

Fat: 11g

Carbohydrates: 30g

Protein: 23g

Veggie Quesadillas with Cilantro Yogurt Dip

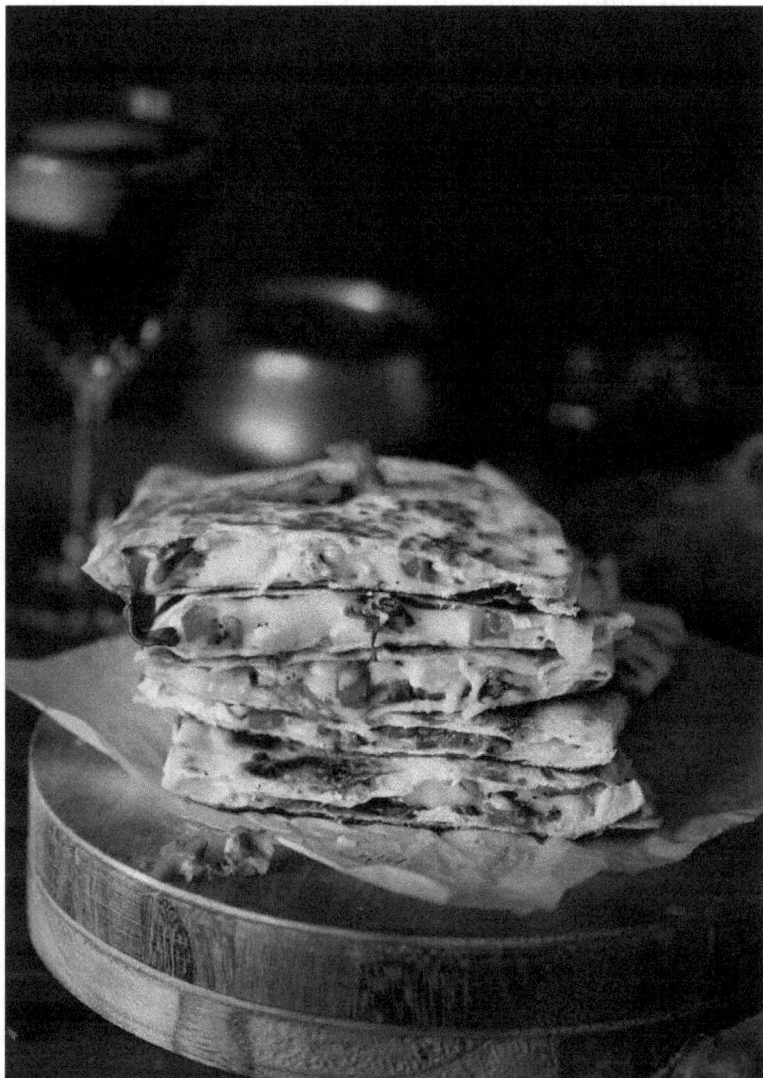

Ingredients

- 1 cup beans, black or pinto

- 2 Tablespoons cilantro, chopped

- ½ bell pepper, finely chopped

- ½ cup corn kernels

- 1 cup low-fat shredded cheese

- Six soft corn tortillas

- One medium carrot, shredded

- ½ jalapeno pepper, finely minced (optional)

- CILANTRO YOGURT DIP

- 1 cup plain nonfat yogurt

- 2 Tablespoons cilantro, finely chopped

- Juice from ½ of a lime

Instructions

1.   Preheat large skillet over low heat.

2.   Line up three tortillas. Spread cheese, corn, beans, cilantro, shredded carrots, and peppers over the tortillas.
3.   Cover all sides with a 2nd tortilla.
4.   Place a tortilla on a dry plate and warmth until cheese is melted and tortilla is slightly golden after 3 minutes.
5.   Flip and cook another side until golden, about 1 minute.
6.   Inside a small bowl, mix the nonfat yogurt, cilantro, and juice.
7.   Cut each quesadilla into four wedges (12 wedges total) and serve three wedges per person with about ¼ cup of the dip.
8.   Refrigerate leftovers within 2 hours.

Yogurt with Almonds & Honey

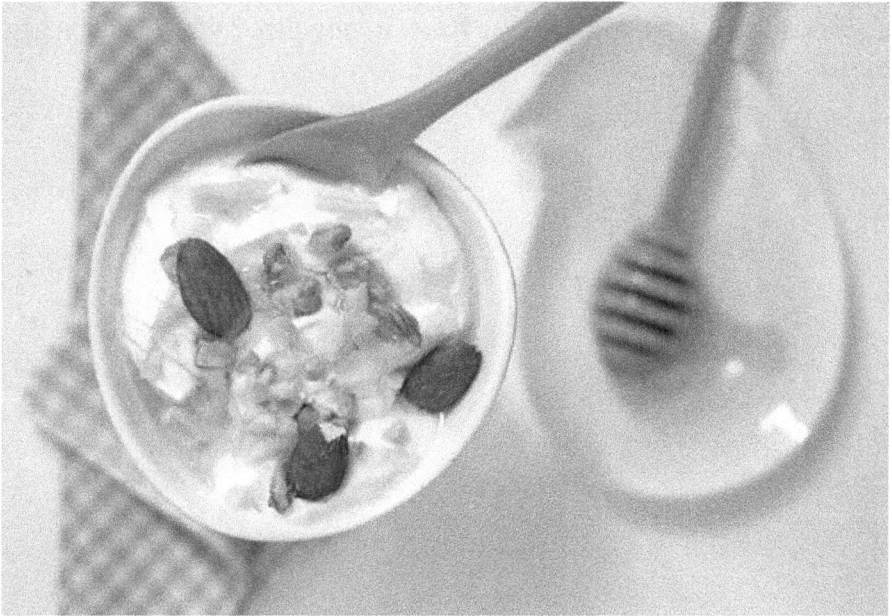

Ingredients

- Non-fat greek yoghurt-Nonfat, plain-16 oz-453 grams

- Almonds-Nuts, raw-1/4 cup, whole-35.8 grams

- Honey-2 tsp-14.1 grams

Directions

Rough-chop almonds and blend into yogurt and honey. Enjoy!

Nutrition

Calories 517 Carbs 36g Fat 20g Protein 54g Fiber 5g Net carbs 31g Sodium 164mg Cholesterol 23mg

Quick Buffalo Chicken Salad

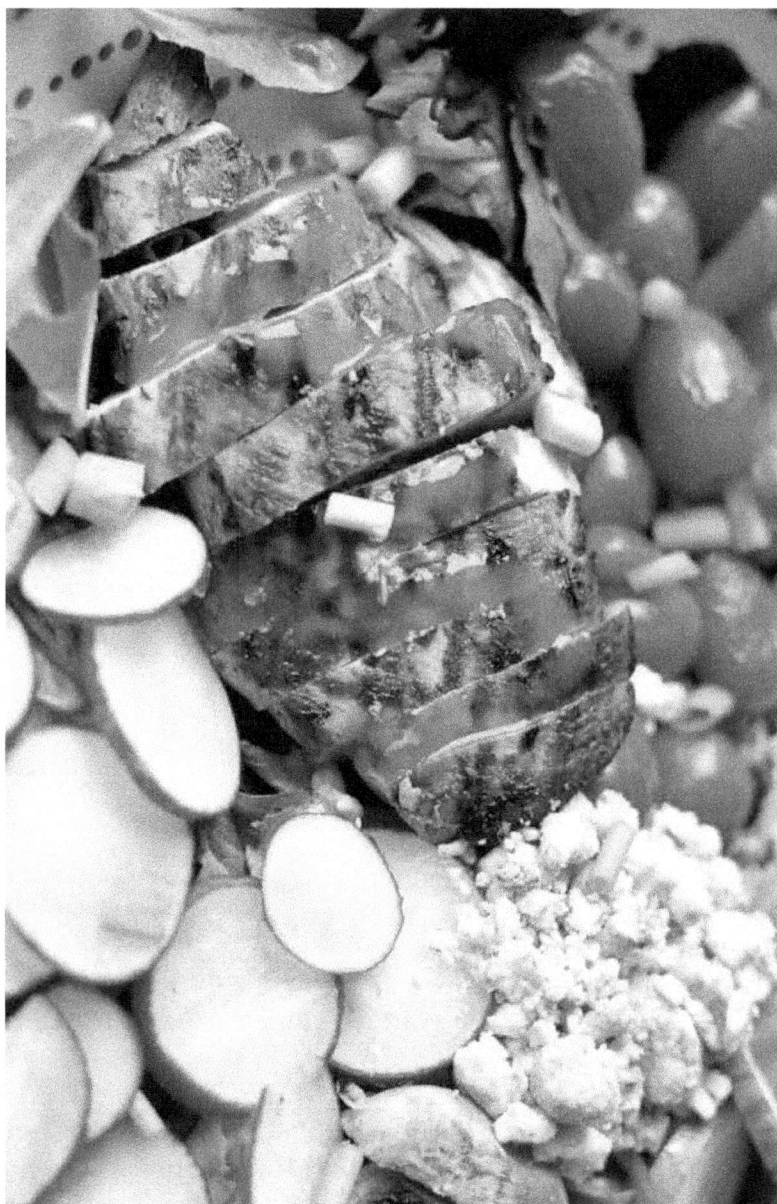

Ingredients

- Pepper or hot sauce-Ready-to-serve-4 tbsp-57.6 grams

- Canned chicken-No broth-1 cup-205 grams

- Spinach-Raw-2 cup-60 grams

- Tomatoes-Green, raw-Two medium-246 grams

Directions

Mix hot sauce with chicken. Spread spinach and tomatoes on the top. Toss together and enjoy it!

Nutrition

Calorie 456 Carbs 18g Fat 18g Protein 57g Fiber 4g Net carbs 13g Sodium 2590mg Cholesterol 103mg

All American Tuna

Ingredients

Tuna-Fish, light, canned in water, drained solids-Two can-330 grams

Light mayonnaise-Salad dressing, light-2 tbsp-30 grams Celery-Cooked, boiled, drained, without a salt-1/4 cup, diced-37.5 grams

Pickles-Cucumber, dill or kosher dill-One large (4" long)-135 grams

Wheat bread-Two slice-50 grams Directions

1. Mix all ingredients in a bowl.

2. Serve with bread.

Nutrition

Calories 512 Carbs 32g Fat 12g Protein 71g Fiber 4g Net carbs 28g Sodium 2443mg Cholesterol 124mg

Pimento Cheese Sandwich

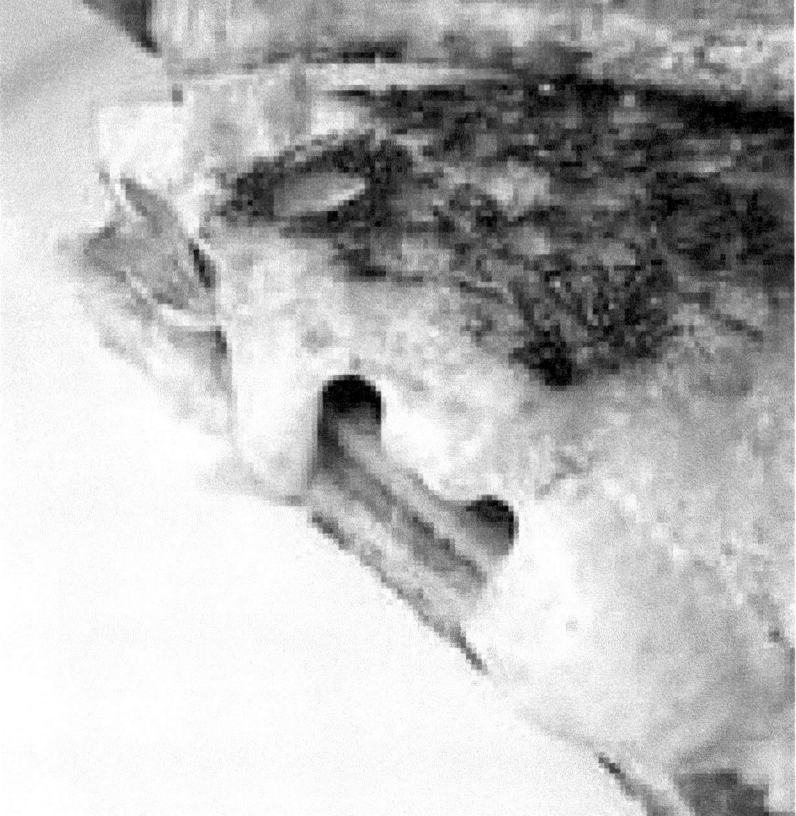

Ingredients

- Pimento cheese-Pasteurized process-2 oz-56.7 grams
- Multi-grain bread-Four slices regular-104 grams

Directions

1. Spread the pimento cheese over the bread.

2. Then, a slice of bread to form a sandwich. Enjoy!

Nutrition

Calories 488 Carbs 46g Fat 22g Protein 26g Fiber 8g Net carbs 38g Sodium 915mg Cholesterol 53mg

Coconut Oil Fat Bombs

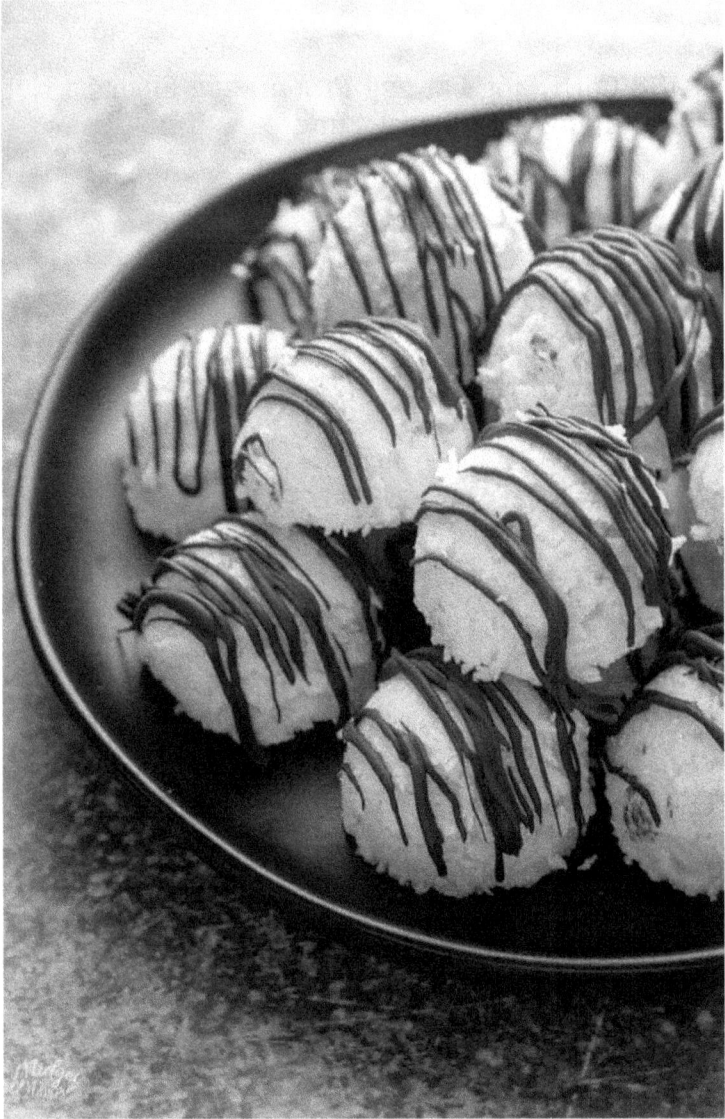

Ingredients

- Coconut oil-1 1/2 tbsp-20.8 grams

- Cocoa-Dry powder, unsweetened-3/4 tbsp-4.1 grams

- Honey-5/16 tsp-2 grams

- Salt-Table-1/8 tsp-0.57 grams

Directions

1.   Mix all the ingredients during a processor until the mixture is smooth and creamy.

2.   Pour into small-sized cube trays or silicone moulds and freeze.

3.   Once frozen, pop the copra oil fat bombs out of the pictures and store them during a freezer zip-top bag or jar. Enjoy!

Nutrition

Calories 194 Carbs 4g Fat 21g Protein 1g Fiber 2g Net carbs 3g Sodium 222mg Cholesterol 0mg

Apricot Jam and Almond Butter Sandwich

Ingredients

Multi-grain bread-Two slices regular-52 grams Jams and preserves-1 tbsp-20 grams

Almond butter-Nuts, every day, without salt, added-1 tbsp-16 grams

Directions

1.   Toast the bread optionally.

2.   Spread almond butter on one side and jam on the other side.

Nutrition

Calories 292 Carbs 39g Fat 11g Protein 10g Fiber 6g Net carbs 34g Sodium 206mg Cholesterol 0mg

Peanut Butter and Honey Toast

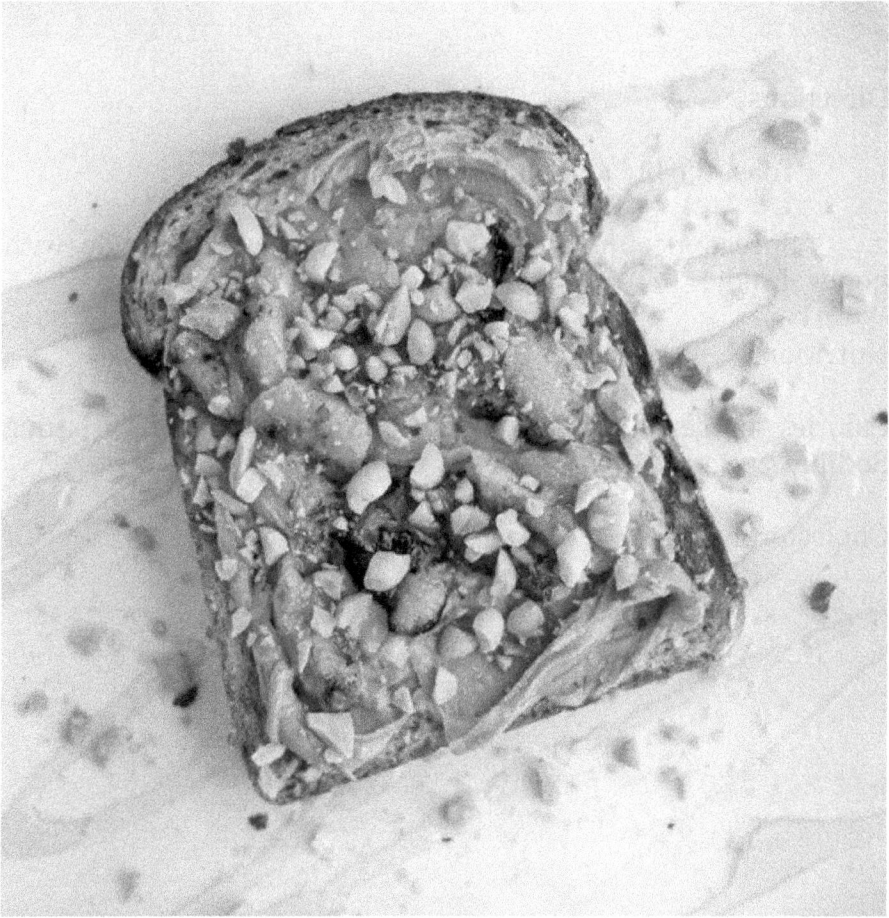

Ingredients

- Multi-grain bread-Two slices regular-52 grams

- Peanut butter-Smooth style, without salt-3 tbsp-48 grams

- Honey-2 tbsp-42 grams

Directions

1.   Toast the bread, and it is optionally.

2.   Spread peanut butter on the bread and sprinkle with honey. Enjoy!

Nutrition

Calories 553 Carbs 68g Fat 27g Protein 18g Fiber 6g Net carbs 62g Sodium 208mg

Cholesterol 0mg

Cucumber & Hummus

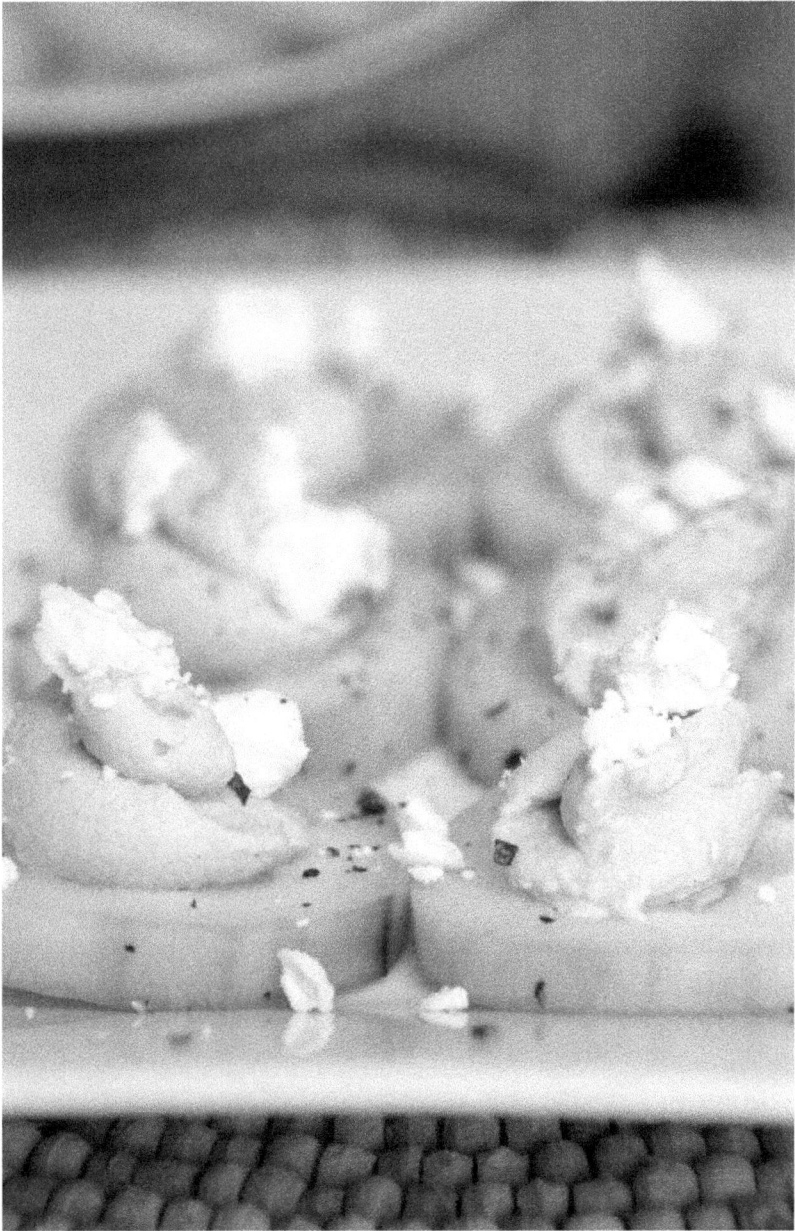

Ingredients

- Hummus-Commercial-1/4 cup-61.5 grams
- Cucumber-With peel, raw-1 cup slices-104 grams

Directions

Cut the cucumber into round slices and eat with hummus.

Nutrition

Calories 118

Carbs13g

Fat6g

Protein6g

Fiber4g

Net carbs8g

Carrot and Hummus Snack

Ingredients

Hummus-Commercial-2 tbsp-30 grams Baby carrots-Baby, raw-1 cup-246 grams

Directions

Dip carrots into hummus and enjoy!

Nutrition

Calories136Carbs25gFat3gProtein4gFiber9gNet

carbs16gSodium306mgCholesterol0mg

Yogurt with Walnuts & Honey

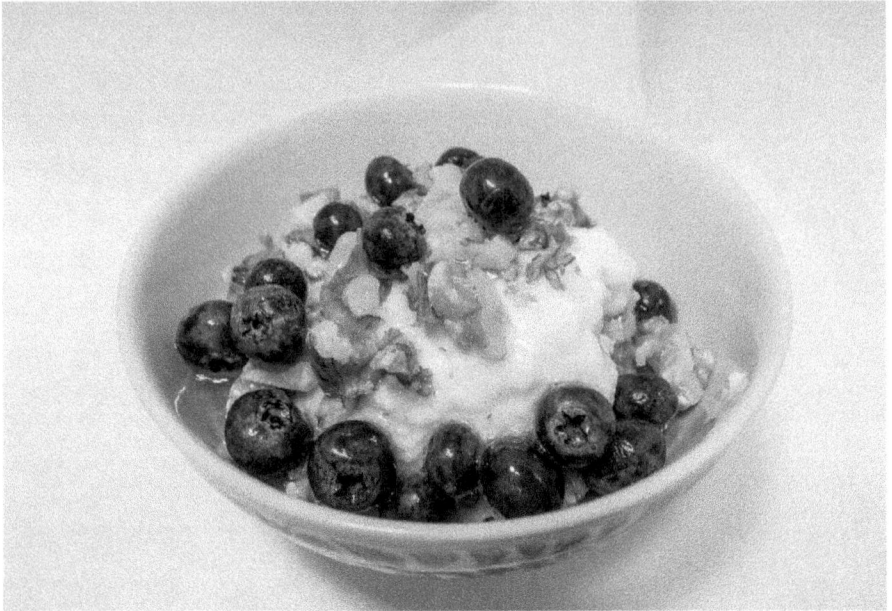

Ingredients

- Walnuts-Nuts, black, dried-1/4 cup, chopped-31.3 grams

- Non-fat greek yoghurt-Nonfat, plain-480cup-480 grams

- Honey-2 tsp-14.1 gram

Directions

1.   Rough-chop walnuts and mix into yogurt.

2.   Top with honey and enjoy!

Nutrition

Calories520Carbs32gFat20gProtein56gFiber2gNet

carbs30gSodium174mgCholesterol24mg

Simple Caprese Sandwich

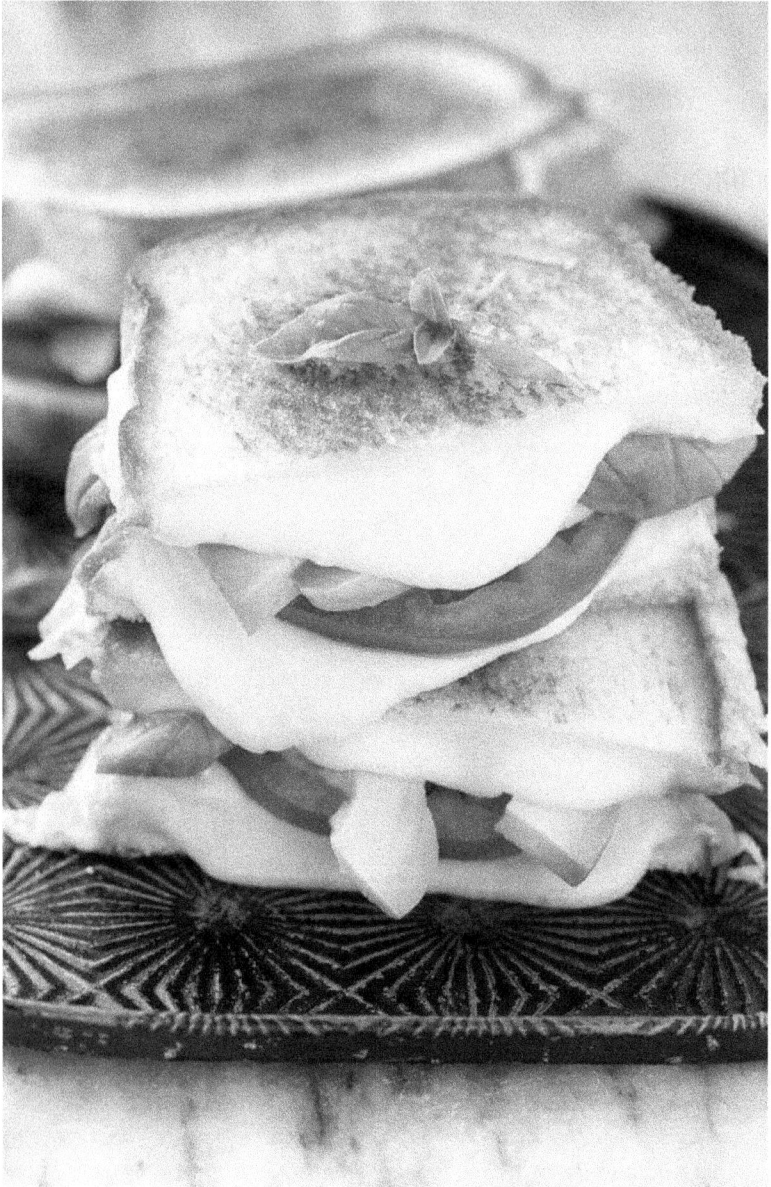

Ingredients

- Sourdough bread, French or Vienna, Two slices, 192 grams Mozzarella cheese

- Whole milk 2 oz 56.7 grams

- Tomatoes - Red, ripe, raw, year-round average

- Four slices, medium (1/4" thick)

Instructions

Cut a large slice of sourdough in half (or use two small slices). Top one slice with 1oz of sliced mozzarella and then two slices of tomatoes. The flavor is mild, so season with salt pepper if desired.

Nutrition

Calories707Carbs104gFat17gProtein34gFiber5gNet

carbs99gSodium1515mgCholesterol45mg

Cottage Cheese Honey Toast

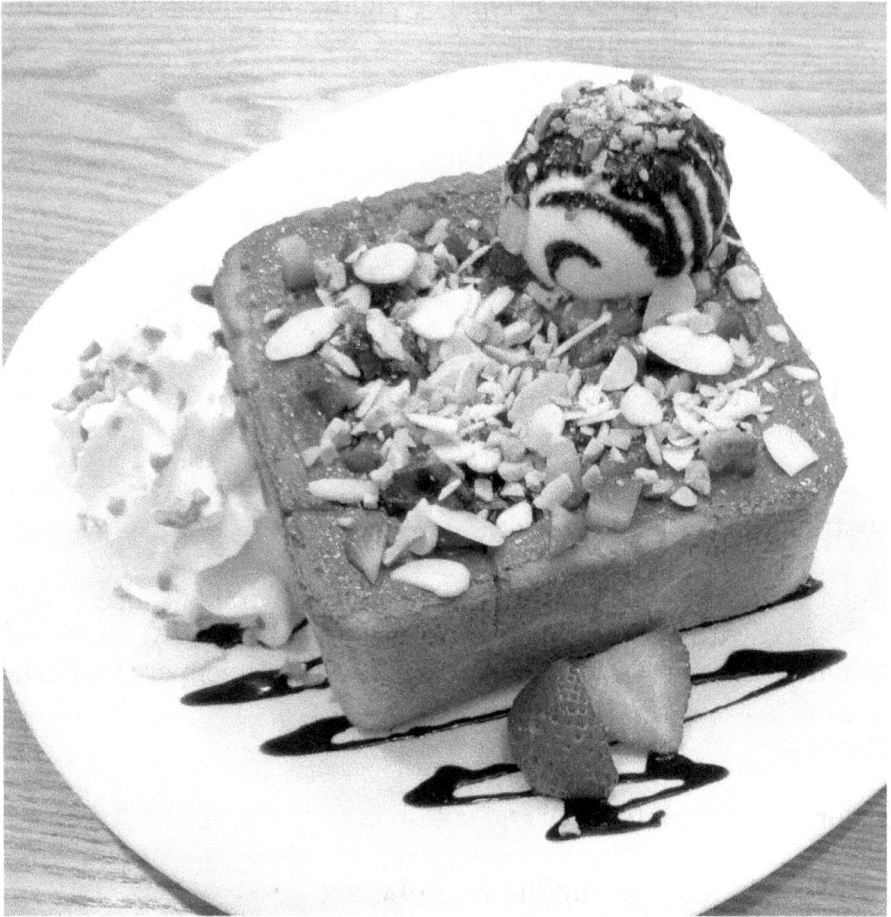

Ingredients

- Whole-wheat bread-Commercially prepared-
- Two slice-56 grams

Cottage cheese- 1% milkfat-1 cup, (not packed)-226 grams

Honey-2 tbsp-42 grams

Directions

Toast bread to your liking. Spread with cottage cheese and drizzle with honey. Enjoy!

Nutrition

Calories432Carbs65gFat4gProtein35gFiber3gNet

carbs61gSodium1174mgCholesterol9mg

Pimento Cheese Sandwich

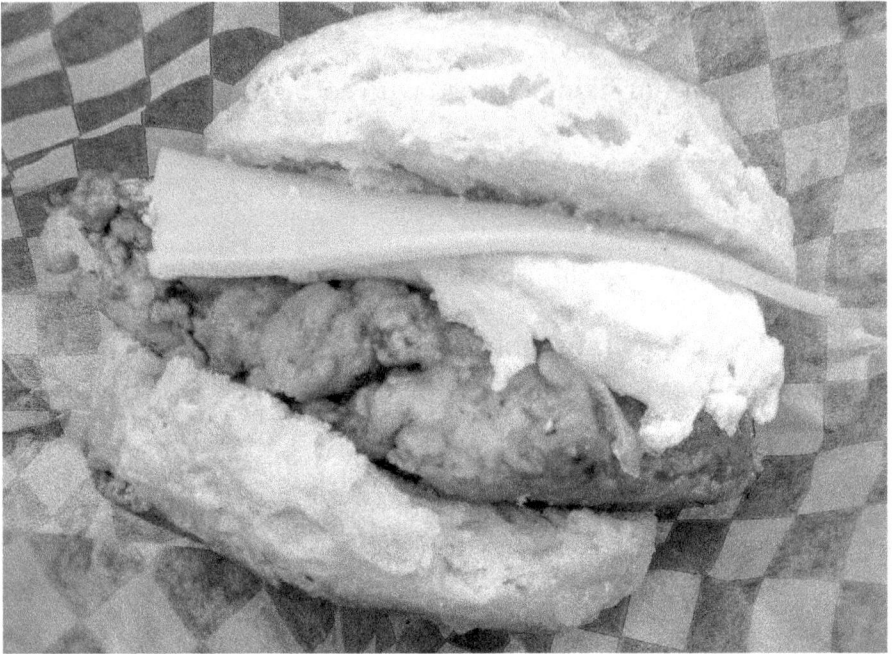

Ingredients

- Pimento cheese-Pasteurized process-2 oz-56.7 grams

- Multi-grain bread-Four slices regular-104 grams

Directions

1.　　Spread the pimento cheese on each side of bread.

And then on the other slice of bread to form a sandwich. Enjoy!

Nutrition

Calories488Carbs46gFat22gProtein26gFiber8gNet
carbs38gSodium915mgCholesterol53mg

Tomato Salad

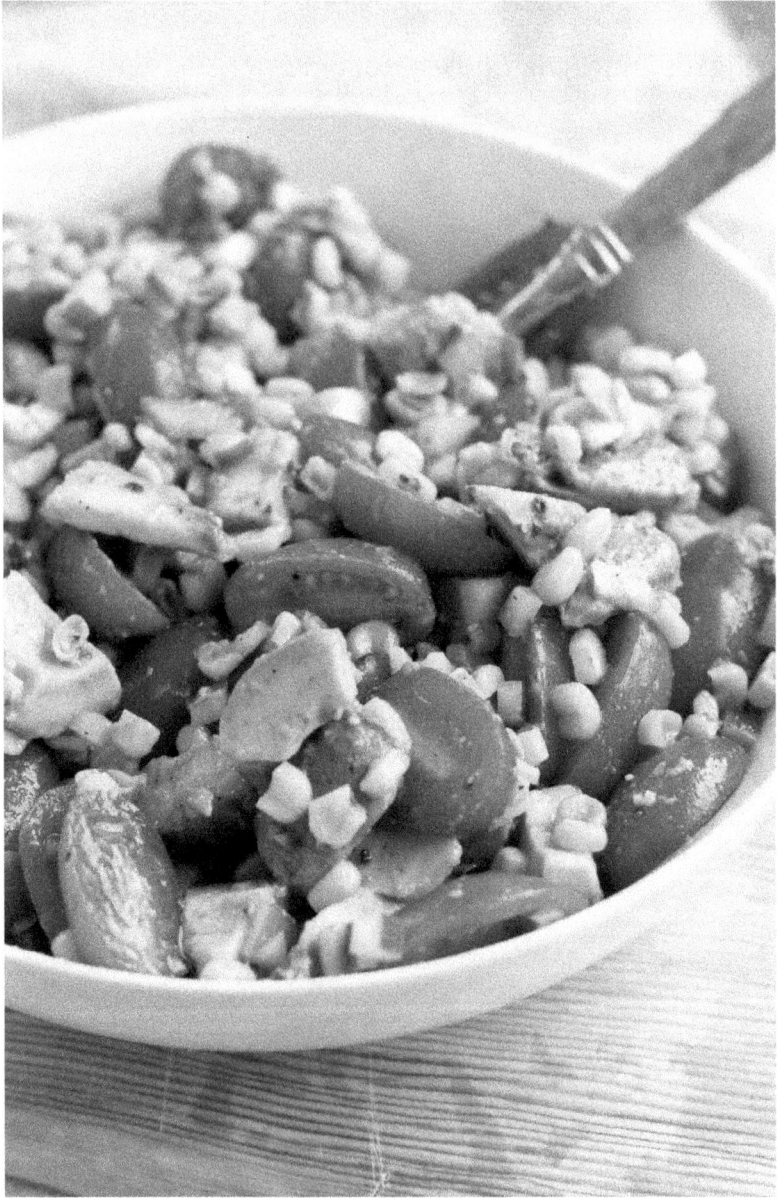

Ingredients

- Vinegar-Cider-2 2/3 tbsp-39.4 grams

- Cucumber-Peeled, raw-Two medium-402 grams

- Onions-Raw-1/2 large-75 grams

- Tomatoes-Red, ripe, fresh, year-round average

- Three medium whole (2-3/5" dia)-369 grams

- Water-Plain, clean water-1/2 cup-118 grams

Directions

Peel and slice cucumbers into coins. Cut tomatoes into pieces. Dice red onion. Add vinegar and water and mix well.

Nutrition

Calories153Carbs31gFat1gProtein6gFiber9gNet

carbs22gSodium32mgCholesterol0mg

Tomato and Cheese Wrap

Ingredients

- Tortillas-2 tortilla -92 grams

- mayonnaise-like dressing-Regular, with salt-2 tbsp-29.4 grams

- Tomatoes-Two medium whole -246 grams

- Lettuce-2 cup shredded-144 grams

- Cheddar cheese-2 oz-56.7 grams

Directions

1. Lightly spread mayo on tortilla shell.

2. Cut tomatoes however you like them.

3. Layer ingredients, spreading them over the tortilla.

4. Tuck up about an inch the side of the shell you've decided is the bottom and roll up the wrap. Enjoy!

Nutrition

Calories638Carbs66gFat32gProtein25gFiber7gNet

carbs59gSodium1236mgCholesterol63mg

Peanut butter yogurt

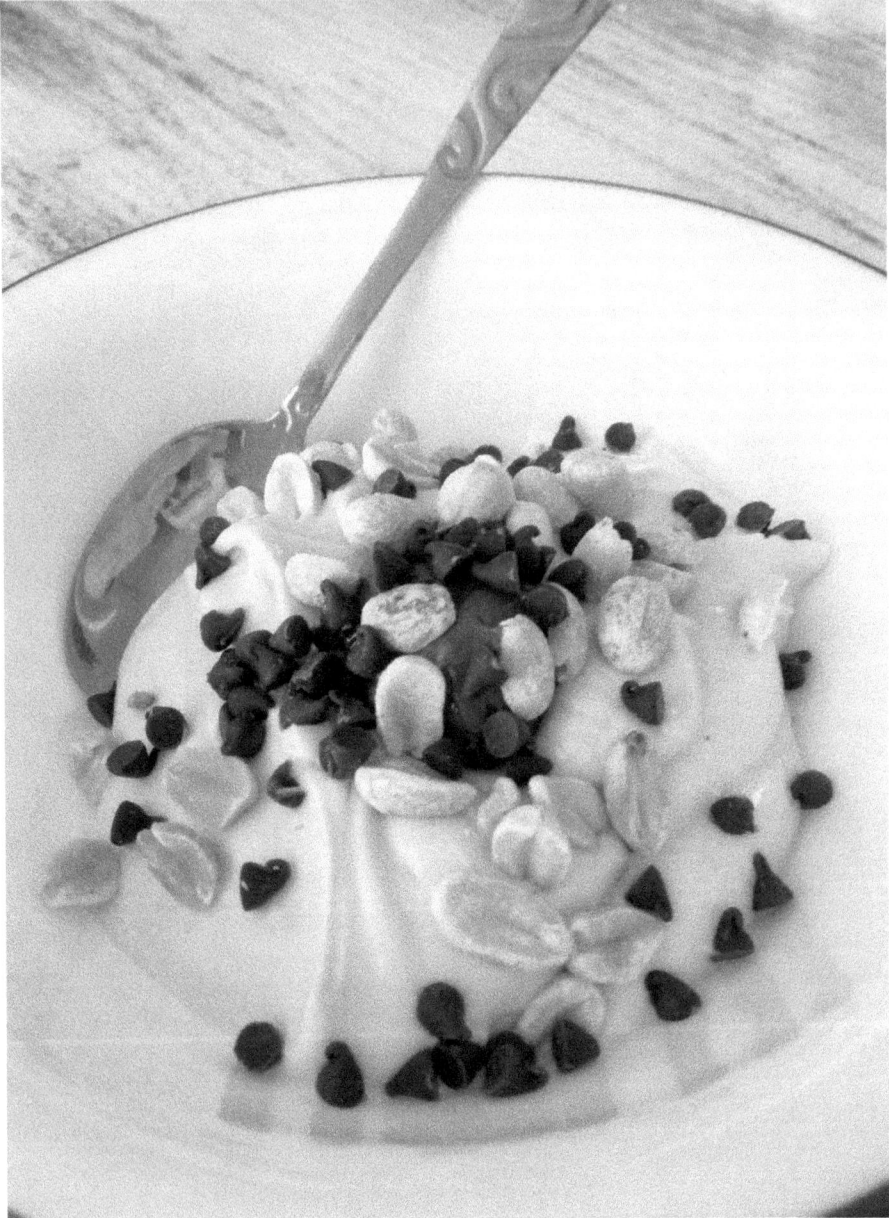

Ingredients

- Nonfat greek yogurt-1 cup-240 grams

- Peanut butter-2 tbsp-32 grams

- Vanilla extract-1 tsp-2.2 grams

Directions

Combine ingredients and enjoy it!

Nutrition

Calories345Carbs16gFat17gProtein32gFiber2gNet

carbs15gSodium223mgCholesterol12mg

Peanut Butter & Carrots

Ingredients

Peanut butter-4 tbsp-64 grams

Carrots-2 cup chopped-256 grams

Directions

Spread peanut butter on carrots and enjoy!

Nutrition

Calories482Carbs38gFat33gProtein18gFiber12gNet carbs26gSodium188mgCholesterol0mg

Cucumber Tomato Salad with Tuna

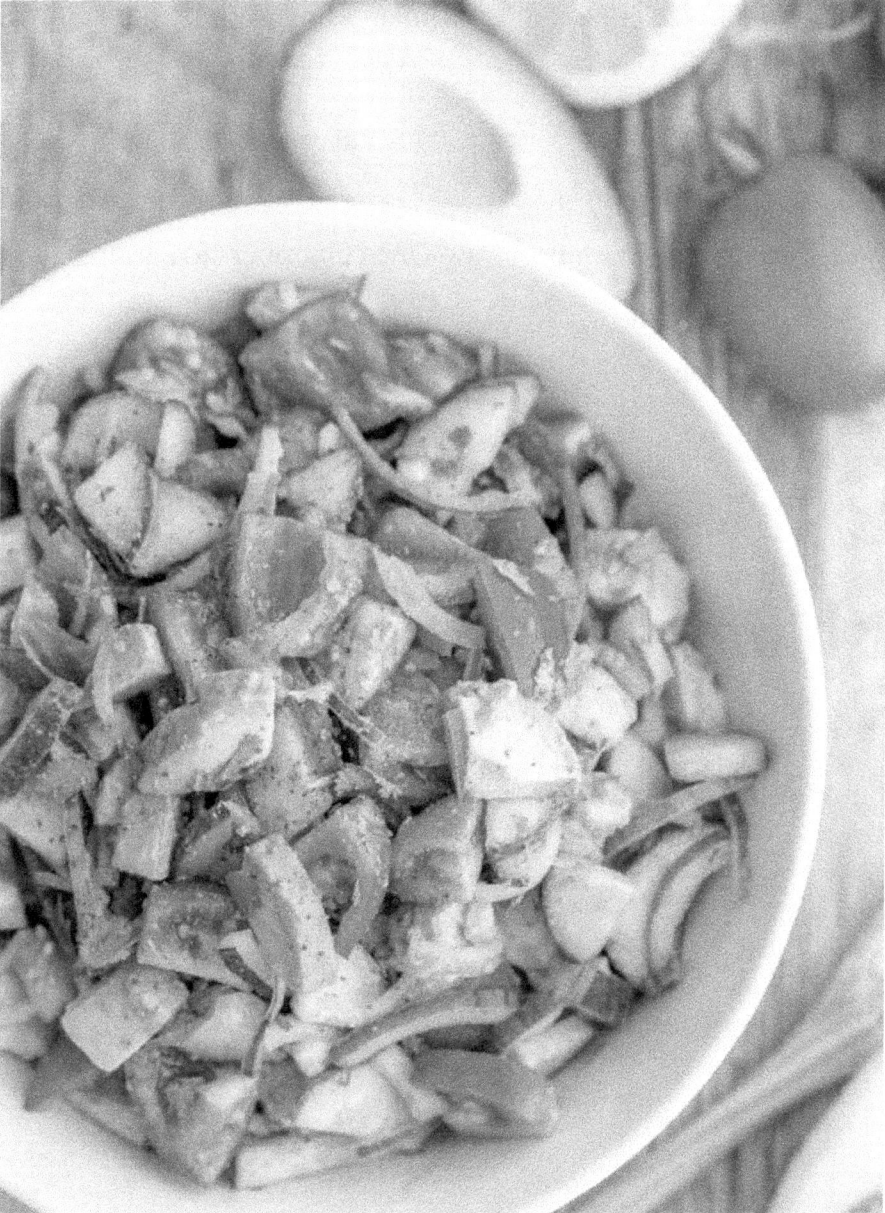

Ingredients

- Tomatoes-Two medium whole -246 grams

- Lettuce-1 cup shredded-36 grams

- Cucumber-With peel, raw-One cucumber-301 grams

- Tuna-One can-165 grams

Directions

1. Chop vegetables and lettuce.

2. Toss together with the tuna and enjoy it!

Nutrition

Calories237Carbs22gFat2gProtein37gFiber5gNet carbs17gSodium436mgCholesterol59mg

Peanut butter and Jelly

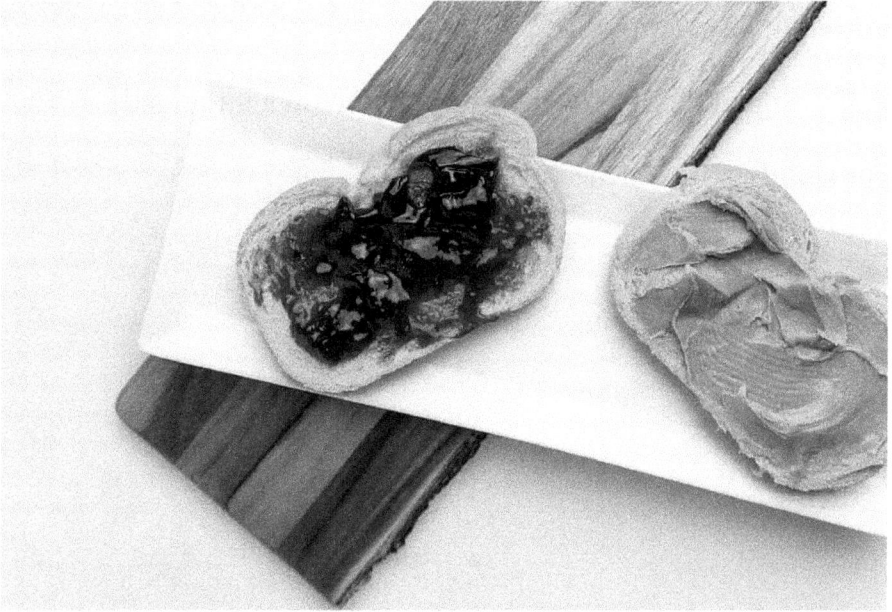

Ingredients

- Multi-grain bread-Four slices regular-104 grams

- Butter-Unsalted-2 tsp-9.5 grams

- Peanut butter-Smooth style, without salt-3 tbsp-48 grams

- Jams and preserves-2 tbsp-40 grams

Directions

1.   Toast the bread, and it's optionally. Drizzle1/2 teaspoon of butter on all sides of the bread.

2.   Spread butter on one side and jam on another side.

Nutrition

Calories742Carbs83gFat37gProtein25gFiber11gNet

carbs73gSodium418mgCholesterol20mg

Chicken Scampi Pasta

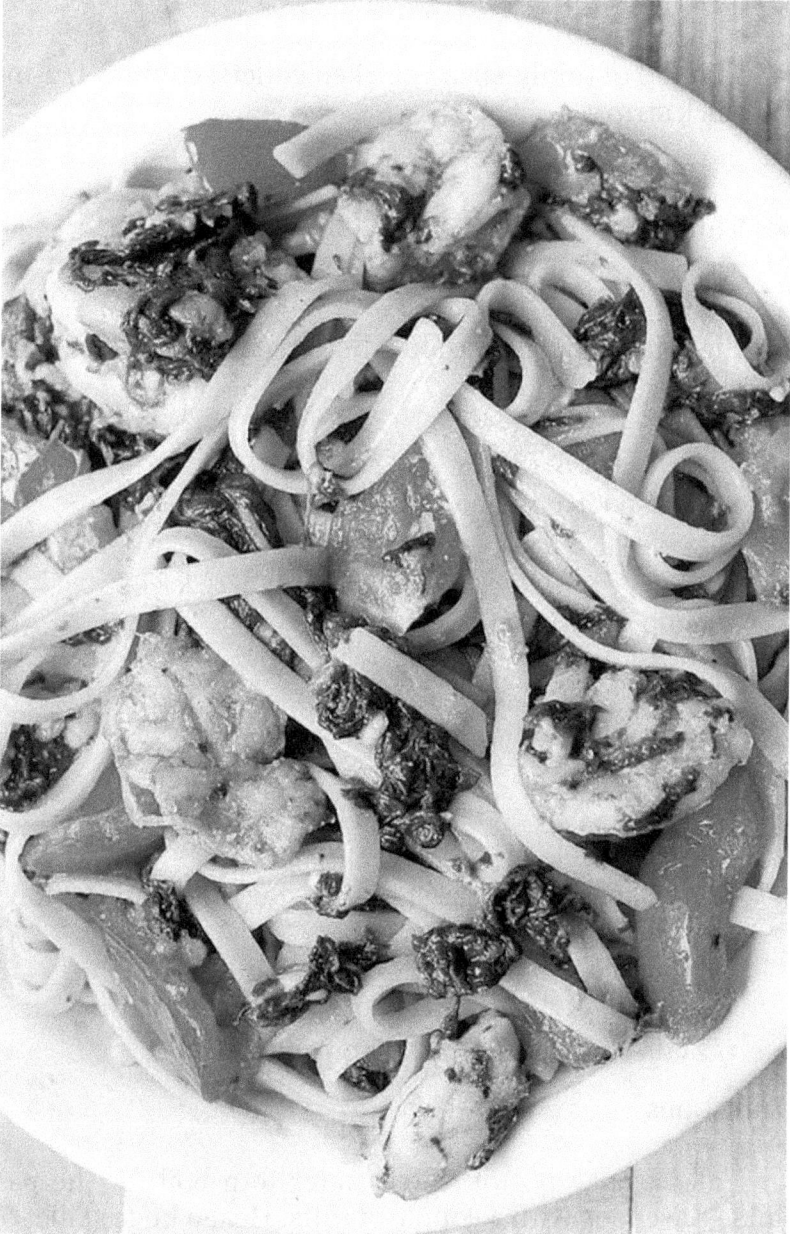

Ingredients

- 1 pound of thinly-sliced chicken cutlets, cut into 1/2-inch-thick strips

- Three tablespoons olive oil

- Eight tablespoons unsalted butter, cubed Six cloves garlic, sliced

- 1/2 teaspoon crushed red pepper flakes

- 1/2 cup dry white wine

- 12 ounces angel hair pasta

- One teaspoon lemon zest plus the juice of 1 large lemon 1/2 cup freshly grated Parmesan

- 1/2 cup chopped fresh Italian parsley

Directions

1.   Take a huge pot of salted water to a boil for the pasta. Sprinkle the chook with a couple of salts. Heat a huge skillet over medium-high warmth until hot, then upload the oil. Working in

2 batches, brown the chook until golden however not cooked through, 2 to a couple of minutes keep with batch. Remove the chicken to a plate.

2.   Melt four tablespoons of the butter within the skillet. Add the garlic and crimson pepper flakes and cook dinner until the garlic begins to show golden at the sides , 30 seconds to 1 minute. Add the wine, deliver to a simmer, and cook dinner till reduced by using half, approximately 2 minutes. Remove from the heat .

3.   Meanwhile, cook dinner the pasta till very hard , reserving 1 cup of the pasta water. Add the pasta and 3/four cup pasta water to the skillet alongside the hen, lemon peel and juice, and therefore the last four tablespoons butter. Return the skillet to medium-low warmness and gently stir the pasta until the butter is melted, including the last word 1/four pasta water if the pasta appears too dry. Remove the skillet from the heat, sprinkle with the cheese and parsley and toss before serving.